WARRIORS!

INSPIRATIONAL STORIES OF WOMEN WHO FOUGHT TO FIND THEIR HEALING

PRINTED IN THE UNITED STATES OF AMERICA

ISBN: 978-0-578-87800-3

Book Cover Design by Rose Miller
Book Cover Photography by Robert Delk III

DEDICATION

To my warriors, my grandmother and mother, thank you for demonstrating strength, power, resiliency, love, respect, and wisdom. Thank you for supporting me and loving me in all, through all, and despite all. Thank you for your sacrifices and dedication. You are truly phenomenal women.

To all of the women around the world, you are enough. You were enough yesterday. You are enough today. You will be enough tomorrow. Wake up each day and strive to be the best version of whom you were called to be. Be true to who you are, understanding that all you need is within you. Be inspired! Be great! Be awesome! Be you! Why? Because the world needs you. You are a warrior!

CONTENTS

THE WAR

Introduction

As women, we navigate a world in which we feel judged, belittled, ostracized, unheard, unvalued, unloved, unprotected, and inadequate. We navigate a world in which our identity and reality collides and we become unrecognizable blank facades. We navigate a world in which being one's authentic self is open to scrutiny and endless debate.

Now imagine adding the intersection of race, class, and gender. Intersectionality, a term introduced by Kimberlé Crenshaw, is used to explore Black women's marginalization (Carbado et al., 2013). Black women often experience the complexity of living at the intersection of multiple marginalized identities, such as being Black, being a woman, and sometimes having a lower socioeconomic status (Spates et al., 2019). The intersection of race, class, and gender often contributes to Black women's health outcomes.

To gain a better understanding of how intersectionality influences the lives of Black women, the following interviews were conducted. Although all of the women were asked the same interview questions, their stories are unique, candid, and raw.

This book highlights the inspirational stories of these 15 incredible Black women who fought to find their healing. Their stories explore how the intersection of race, class, and gender has influenced their lives. As they share their stories and allow us into their lives, they demonstrate bravery, strength, and resiliency. They are warriors!

A WAR OF IDENTITY

A Warrior Named Jo:
Her Battle with Sexual Identity

Color outside the lines.
—Jo

Society often tries to dictate who we are, who we should be, how we should behave, and what gender roles we should play. But what happens when who we are does not align with who society tells us we should be?

Herein, Jo, a 31-year-old married Black woman, discusses her sexuality, sexual identity, gender roles, and labels. Let's dive in.

Her Definition

Sexuality is defined as fluid and constantly evolving.

As defined by Alexander et al. (2017), sexuality refers to an individual's sexual and romantic attraction to other individuals.

Her Experience

My weight and the fact that I am often typecast as a *stud* influence how I navigate the world. I think people associate sexuality with your size and visual representation. As your weight increases, the only clothing options available are the grandma flower dresses.

On top of that, I had to navigate how to *come out*. It seemed as though everyone had a coming out story, but I didn't. I was very laid back when I came out. I told my mother at Red Lobster. I didn't feel the need to have an elaborate event or anything like that.

Then, the day after my mom passed away, November 29, 2013, I woke up and thought, *Oh, hell no. Fuck these labels because they will not get you anywhere.* When you allow people to label you, you allow them to establish your value. That's not something I'm willing to do. When someone says, "Oh, you're a stud," then I will have to fall privy to society's stud-like tendencies and behaviors. No, I'm Jo, and I don't have time for labels.

I like to wear hats, but I also like to make sure my hair is done and I have earrings to go with the hat. I also like getting my eyebrows threaded, a manicure, and a pedicure. However, I also love my sweatpants. I make the outfit; the outfit doesn't make me.

Her Well-Being

By not identifying with sexual labels, I get to break all the rules. I'm cool enough to be with the guys, but I'm also cool enough to hang with the sisters. It's an enigma, and I get pleasure out of being able to walk that fine line. I use my sexuality as a badge of honor. Sometimes I want to say, "Do you know what I've been through? Sweetheart, no. I was homosexual before this shit was cool!"

While I get pleasure out of being able to walk that line emotionally, it can be draining. Sometimes, the guys forget that I'm a woman. When I respond like a woman, they are sometimes shocked, like, "Oh, you are a girl." Then, when I'm with my girls, they'll tell me what guys are saying. I respond, "Nope. I promise you missed something. That's not what he said." It's an uphill journey that takes years to figure out and can be emotionally exhausting.

It's been one hell of a ride, honestly. I grew up in the church. My grandmother was in the Church of God in Christ Pentecostal, and my mom grew up Baptist. When I first came out, I thought I couldn't love God and be gay. I felt like I couldn't be saved because I was taught that if you're gay, you're going to hell. At the same time, I was taught that those going to hell don't believe in Jesus. To show belief in Jesus, you have to confess with your mouth, believe in your heart, and accept Jesus as your Savior to have eternal life. I did that—all of it. So, I was conflicted. I had to dig deep within myself to determine what I believed in. Once I dug deep, I began to question the entire structure of what I was taught because this was not a religion I picked—I was born into it.

I began studying other religions, reading the Quran, studying Buddhism, Judaism, and more. It was then that I realized that as Christians, if we say God is the Alpha and Omega, then He should be able to stand the test of time. I then realized the purpose of religion is to become the best version of yourself.

When you are gay in a heteronormative society, you cannot move in any direction. You have to proceed straight until told or shown otherwise. It was draining because I was trying to fit into a box that did not fit me.

That conflict caused me to eat my feelings. I ate everything—from German chocolate cake to carrot cake to pound cake. Food was my comfort. Looking back, I'm grateful for the experience because it allowed me to harness my emotions and transform them into a profitable business. Dealing with my emotions taught me how to turn the bad into good—you know, make lemonade out of lemons.

So now when I think of not identifying with sexual labels, I think of boundaries, rules, and limits—boundaries people impose on you because they think they can tell you what you can and cannot do. You don't know me. Who says I can't do it? Why can't I do it?

With rules, everyone has their ideas of who I am and what I should be, what I can and cannot do, and what I should believe. People believe me and my wife are not straight enough, and others say we're not gay enough. For example, the gay community considers my wife and I too straight. We do not identify with all the pronouns, so that caused issues. I didn't even know what a stud was until about a year and a half ago. Again, I wasn't living by labels.

Finally, I think of limits because you can't limit me. You can't tell someone to be their authentic self and live in their authentic truth but only if it fits a heteronormative society. I feel like Black women will never fit in. Our authentic selves don't fit what America says is authentic. Can you imagine being a Black woman who already does not fit in, then adding another layer such as being plus size, and then on top of that being someone who does not identify with sexual labels?

That being said, I compare not identifying with sexual labels to the Civil Rights Movement. I remember in the early 2000s, Ellen DeGeneres said that being gay was the new Black. It caused an uproar in the Black community. However, it was true because we had to fight for our rights. As Blacks, we had to fight for our right to vote and to go to desegregated schools, and it's the same for the LGBTQA+ community. We had to fight for marriage and fight for shared health insurance. If we were all equal, the process would be the same for all people, regardless of our sexuality.

Her Support System

My support system was a party of one—my best friend in college. I remember when I was a freshman and telling her how I felt. She was a psychology major, so I felt comfortable talking to her. She created a peaceful and comfortable atmosphere, which is what I needed.

I didn't know how to tell my mother. It's not because I feared that she would not love me anymore; it was because we were close. It's crazy because people think the number one fear someone has when they come out is someone not loving you anymore, but the fear is people changing how they are around us. They say, "Oh, she's living that lifestyle." But sweetie, our lives are no different from anyone else's; we happen to lie with someone of the same gender. Some people take homosexuality as a reason to treat us differently. What could be so repulsive that you have the right to mistreat someone who chooses to love and be involved with someone of the same gender?

Overall, my support system was beneficial. I had a counselor and my best friend, who was my pillar of support. I also had my mom. She disagreed with my lifestyle, but she had my back, and that's what I needed.

However, looking back, I wish I was not secretive about my sexuality. I wish the 24-year-old me would have known I was going to be this way. I've matured to the point where I don't care what others think. I will not give others the power to label me. If I allow you to label me, I've given you the power to control me.

Her Intersection of Healthcare

For people like me, the healthcare system is as difficult to navigate as anywhere else. When my wife got sick, the hospital staff didn't treat me the same way they would have treated a heterosexual couple. If I were a man, they would have praised me for staying by my wife's side and advocating for her when she couldn't do so for herself. However, as a woman in a relationship with another woman, I was told, "Not right now" or "We don't have time." I had to talk to the hospital chairperson to get things in motion. Only when I started making statements about discriminatory practices was I taken seriously. It shouldn't be like that.

Additionally, when I went to the hospital for my weight loss surgery, they asked, "What is your pronoun?" It was the first time I've ever heard that in my life. Some of what I experienced seemed so advanced and unnecessary. I'm not Jo the lesbo. I'm Jo.

Her Healing

I was able to cope with not identifying with sexual labels because I have a policy with everyone: if you don't know, ask. There's no offense if the questions or statements come from a genuine place of interest or concern.

However, my biggest challenge in not identifying with sexual labels was balance. Balance is hard because we live in a world where things are black and white. That is not easy because I live in a very colorful world. We allow people to choose their gender as nonbinary, but we don't allow people to choose their sexuality. I do not fit within the lines. I become the outlier.

When people see me—if I'm sitting down—they assume I'm a guy. However, when I stand, they realize I am a woman. I have to be especially mindful as a Black woman, specifically in how I orate, because I don't want to be seen as an angry Black woman. It's always a balance of asserting myself without appearing to be dominant and angry.

However, I can say that my greatest triumph has been self-awareness. I am completely free. The funny thing in my turning point with not identifying with sexual labels was when my wife and I had a double date with a lesbian couple. During the date, one of the women kept referring to the other woman as "her husband." I was a little confused at first, but then I thought, "All right, this is how we're rolling." The woman who was being referred to as the husband thought that I was a stud. She mentioned, "You know how we studs do." I'm like, "No, I don't."

Thinking back over my journey, I would tell my younger self not to worry about other people's opinions. I would also tell my younger self to "control your life to control the game because he who controls the game makes the rules." That's why I would tell other women to be 100% themselves because tomorrow is not promised. You have to love yourself for yourself and realize that you are enough. What you say to yourself and about yourself matters. It's like looking in a mirror. I realize that it has been 10 years since I made this decision. I can't wait for the next 10 years.

Now, let's analyze in depth Jo's story to gain an understanding of her refusing to identify with sexual labels. In her closing remarks, Jo made it clear that she's striving to be her best self, live in her truth, and not be subjected to other's labels. I praise Jo for controlling her narrative and not giving others the power to define her. I also commend Jo for taking a stand and understanding her worth is not based on her sexual identity and visual appearance.

Although identities are not additive because oppression is about one's experiences, I am reminded that Black women who do not identify with sexual labels experience "triple jeopardy," a term coined by Beverly Green. Triple jeopardy encompasses the barriers Black nonheterosexual women experience due to living in a society that devalues people who are of color, women, and sexual minorities (Cerezo et al., 2020). Thus, intersecting oppressions (Black, woman, and does not identify with sexual labels) are woven through multiple identities and interconnected experiences. These interconnected identities can result in consequences, especially when we assess this country's historical context regarding Blacks, women, and those who do not identify with labels.

That being said, I applaud Jo for seeking wholeness by diving deeper into her spirituality, seeking counseling, and not allowing others to label her. It takes courage and strength to walk in your truth and be true to yourself. Remember what Jo said: "Take control of the game because he who controls the game makes the rules" and "What you say to yourself and about yourself matters."

We have to remember that there is life and death in the tongue, and there's power in what we tell ourselves each day. We must speak life into ourselves each day, even when society says otherwise. We cannot subscribe to the notion that we have to fit in a box, especially a box that was never meant for us to be in. We are more than that box. We are more powerful than that box. We are worth more than that box. Reclaim your power, sis. You got this. Remember, you are enough, you are powerful, you are valued, and you are loved. Girl, you are a warrior!

A WAR OF CANCER

A Warrior Named Janice:
Her Battle with Breast Cancer

I survived because she (my mom) lives within me. When she died of cancer, I was 11 years old. I was left with her peace, strength, love, resilience, harmony, and hope. These characteristics propelled me to rise from the ashes like the phoenix, and I continue to live because she could not.

—Janice

Among women, breast cancer is the second leading cause of cancer in the United States (Centers for Disease Control and Prevention, 2020a). Although White women and Black women are diagnosed with breast cancer at similar rates, Black women are 40% more likely to die.

Let's turn to a warrior named Janice to gain a better understanding of her experience with breast cancer. Janice is a 41-year-old Black woman. Here is her story.

Her Definition

There are many ways to define breast cancer. However, my personal definition is breast cancer is an invasion to the mind, body, and spirit that plagues women across the world.

Although there are multiple types of breast cancer, the most basic medical definition of breast cancer is a disease in which cells in the breast grow out of control (Centers for Disease Control and Prevention, 2020a).

8

Her Experience

In addition to being a Black woman, other circumstances have influenced how I navigate the world in terms of breast cancer. Since I was young, I have been intimately aware of breast cancer because my mother, in her early 40s, was diagnosed with breast cancer and passed away when I was 11 years old. Other women in my family, like my mother's sister, also had breast cancer. Further, other Black women in my community had breast cancer. At the age of 32, I too was diagnosed with breast cancer. Thus, having intimately witnessed so many women battle breast cancer, I was and am aware of the trauma that breast cancer has on your life.

I became acutely aware that women in my family had a predisposition toward breast cancer due to living in poverty, being Black, and facing racism. In my community, domestic violence also played a role. All of these societal issues predisposed the women in my family toward breast cancer.

When I was diagnosed with breast cancer, I was a full-time doctoral student. I was enrolled in classes and working as a graduate assistant to maintain my student medical insurance. At my university, we had a medical school. Therefore, my student medical insurance gave me access to all the specialists.

My nightmare began when I did a self-exam and felt something weird—a lump. I remember hoping it would go away because sometimes the breasts go through changes. When it didn't go away, I called the nurse who usually does my mammograms, and she got me in right away. The scan came back abnormal, so they opted to do a biopsy. I went to the appointment alone and afraid. The day of the biopsy, my partner and I quarreled, and I was stressed out and questioning the relationship. He was supposed to go to the appointment with me, but I told him not to because I didn't want the extra stress.

When the pathology report came back positive for breast cancer, I felt as if I was in a movie. It was surreal. Who gets breast cancer at the age of 32? I didn't recognize myself anymore. I thought about my future and what life would be like for me. I wanted to make sure I did everything to fulfill my life's purpose, but I also felt sad and selfish because I wanted to live and do the things I wanted to do in life. I was conflicted. What if that is not what God intended for me? My thinking changed completely, and I was sad all the time.

I was a young woman thinking about how breast cancer could affect me. Would I still be fertile? Would I die young like my mom? Would I end up with scars all over my body that would serve as a constant reminder of my battle? I constantly endured those moments of introspection until I had a rising phoenix moment. I felt like a part of who I once was had died, but I reemerged as a survivor. I was diagnosed in 2012 and feel that little of the old me is left from who I was before my diagnosis. I have a lot of new parts that I didn't know were there. The experience was transformational, even though it was at times overwhelmingly bad. Battling breast cancer made me look at life completely differently because when confronted by your mortality, you begin to examine what is most important in life.

Her Well-Being

Before I was diagnosed with breast cancer, I was teaching a trauma class. After my diagnosis, I looked more closely at trauma as it relates to health outcomes. Additionally, I had childhood trauma and historical trauma. On top of everything else, my own diagnosis enhanced my understanding of how people often push through adversities without learning how to properly regulate their emotions due to trauma. I was determined to help people understand the importance of leaving toxic situations that may add to their level of distress and thereby contribute to their trauma. The diagnosis made me more aware of my body and the historical underpinnings of Black women's health and trauma.

The exploration and discovery of these issues led to an increased understanding of Black women as matriarchs who serve within their communities as resources, helpers, comforters, and caretakers. My mother, for instance, was an educator and disciplinarian. She worked full-time, helped my dad in the garden, was a seamstress, and was known in the community as a holistic healer. My illness certainly helped me view my mother in a more appreciative light.

I'm the youngest of four and sometimes viewed as a person who knows much, but this experience reminded me that I know very little. Sometimes I don't have all the answers. There were things in my life that I was trying to navigate through. I navigated what was going on with my body and wondered if I would ever be in another romantic relationship after my partner and I broke up shortly after my treatment. He was the last person to see the old me. There was so much grief and loss. I lost my hair and endured body changes, scars, and much more due to chemotherapy and radiation.

In this hair-shaming culture, my Blackness was questioned because my hair didn't look a certain way. And let's not forget the body-shaming from everyone. Those thoughts, comments, and reactions from others and my own grief combined with the stress I dealt with as a Black woman and cancer survivor. It was challenging because I was really trying to survive. There were many times I just wanted to scream, "Can I live today? It's not about you!"

This world can be so unforgiving. I felt the world's harshness even more because I was a doctoral student working in a highly competitive environment. It hit me a little harder because I couldn't understand the competition. I couldn't understand why anyone would want to compete with me when there's enough room at the table for everyone. The competition, combined with all of the other complexities of life, caused me to keep to myself, cross my T's, dot my I's, and get my work done to keep my job. I look back and wonder how people couldn't see that I was trying to avoid these spaces. I was the only Black woman at work and the only Black woman on tenure track, and I was being taxed by microaggressions. I had to figure out how to maneuver around everything.

I hit rock bottom mentally and emotionally. I built myself up again with God and know I wouldn't be where I am now without Him. Once I got to the point where I understood that breast cancer is neither finite nor infinite, I made up my mind to live. It's not finite as in a death sentence, and it is not infinite in that I would never be in remission. My life is not over. I can be safe but still have a good time. I don't know when my life will end, so I'm going to enjoy all it brings until I cease being on this earth.

Even though I have all of these positive thoughts and feelings about God carrying me through, I still struggle physically. Having breast cancer made me more aware of what I put in my body. I grew up in a rural, impoverished Black community. I didn't realize we were poor because it seemed we had everything we needed and everyone lived on a farm. I now realize that I have more privilege today than I did back then because I get to choose what I eat and am not required to eat whatever is put on the table. I am, however, much more careful about what I consume.

I decided to stop eating meat and cheese, and I took a second look at other foods as well. Being a Black woman, I am predisposed to health issues because of racism/sexism, and being from a rural community also adds to that vulnerability.

This vulnerability often has me reflecting on the day that I found out that I had breast cancer. I can see myself sitting in my car in the parking garage trying to stop crying so that I could drive home. I also think about my mom and the way she struggled with her cancer. Because I was the youngest and often the only one at home with her, I helped her with many tasks she was unable to do for herself. Although those things were hard to do, they represent the last memories I have of her.

One of my own bad experiences that affects me tremendously relates to when I realized my hair was falling out. I didn't want to be too hard on my hair, so I wasn't combing it; I wasn't doing anything. I was rubbing coconut oil on it. Then a beautician at the hospital consulted with me. Our conversation went like this:

She: Is your hair starting to fall out?

Me: No, I still have hair. It's there.

She: Can I see? (Pulls off my hat and gives me a pitying look.) I'm sorry to tell you this, but your hair is literally just barely connected to your head. (I start to cry.)

She: Do I have permission? Can I shave your hair for you?

Thus, there I sat, looking in the mirror, watching this woman shave my hair off, and I just lost it.

Having breast cancer is horrific and beautiful at the same time, kind of like weeds. Although they are thorny and compromising to plants, they still can produce flowers. Breast cancer stayed in me long enough to produce flowers, but then it had to be removed so that the rest of me could grow and thrive.

Her Support System

Even though we had issues beforehand and problems afterward, my partner was all hands on deck during my breast cancer experience. He went to every appointment and took notes. When I was doing chemotherapy, he sat beside the bed and held the bucket as I vomited. He told them what to give me and what not to give me. Although we broke up, I am so grateful that he was there during that moment, during those times, because he was consistent.

My sorority sisters were also part of my support system. During my infusions, one of my sorority sisters who's kind of like my mom would come and read a book. My other sorority sisters would bring me a candle, some lotion, or take me on a walk. Since I had a compromised immune system, they would pick me up and drive me to classes so I wouldn't have to ride the bus.

In addition, a faculty member who was a full professor, a Black woman, a sorority sister, and two-time survivor of breast cancer—and whose mom had breast cancer—would always check in on me. She would give me things such as a book about changing your diet.

My support system was very beneficial. They met me where I was. I never felt like somebody was telling me how to do something. They just let me be. They extended unconditional love.

Her Intersection of Healthcare

Oh, let me tell you how the healthcare system influenced my experience with breast cancer. My oncologist, oh, my goodness. He knew his science, but I remember many microaggressions. When I first started my treatment, I had kinky twists. His assistant said, "Oh, I'm so sorry, you're probably going to lose that beautiful hair you have." My oncologist replied, "Oh, that's not her hair; those are extensions."

In addition, I kept trying to tell him that I was experiencing something psychological when I came to the hospital. As I entered the hospital, I would throw up. He kept trying to prescribe medication to handle it, but the medicine was making me sick. I continued to tell him that it was psychological. He should have recommended a counselor or something to decrease stress; however, he did not make any recommendation until my last chemotherapy infusion. I thought, *Are you kidding me? This is the end of my six-month road; are you for real?* I felt ignored. They were not considerate.

Although I experienced difficult times in the healthcare system, I had positive moments as well. One of my most positive memorable moments in the healthcare system was when I started radiation. I spoke with the radiologist, and I told her that I did not understand how I did not carry the BRCA gene, but my mom, her sister, and later my sister developed breast cancer. She explained it so simply. She said to think of breast cancer as an apple tree. We got the most prominent and shiniest apples (genes) because they were ripe. They were big. They were ready. However, that doesn't mean that there aren't other apples (genes) that can cause cancer. The way she broke that down, it felt like she cared. I appreciated her for taking the time to do that.

Her Healing

I am still coping with breast cancer; it's a lifelong process. When coping strategies failed, which they sometimes do, I developed positive coping strategies. I went to counseling and wrote several light poems. I also started working out. I lost approximately 25–30 pounds.

My biggest challenge was mentally coping with being diagnosed with breast cancer. However, my biggest triumph was being a survivor. The turning point in life was when I hit rock bottom in reference to my mental health. I realized that I needed to change some things. I needed to start reframing and rewriting what I envisioned my future to be.

That's why, looking back, I would tell myself not to eat fast food. I would also tell the younger version of myself not to sweat the small stuff. Focus on what you can control and be your best because your best is always good enough. You don't have to be Superwoman.

My advice for other women who are experiencing breast cancer is that if you don't like your oncologist, get a second opinion and, if possible, switch because hopefully you'll only go through this once. You should at least be comfortable with who is providing your healthcare. Throughout the process, focus on balance. You don't want to ask too many people who experienced breast cancer, "What happened to you? What did you do?" Their plan is going to be different from yours. However, you should have a community of women who may have gone through the process who can give you tips about what to do, what to ease up on, and symptoms. Finally, I would say love yourself and accept the new person that you're becoming. You can view it in one of two ways: you can view the transformation as "I'm losing the person

I used to be and that makes me sad," or you can view it as "I'm gaining a new version of me, and that's beautiful." As I reflect upon where I am today, I'm still developing, I'm still growing. I hope that I continue to grow and do not become stagnant.

Now, let's intimately reflect upon Janice's story, a story of strength and resiliency. Janice spoke about how aware she was of her predisposition toward breast cancer due to her family history with breast cancer, living in poverty, being Black, and facing racism. Janice makes a great point; here's why.

One must not forget, Black and White women are similarly diagnosed with breast cancer, yet Black women are more likely to die. Thirty-one percent of Black women diagnosed with breast cancer will not survive (Breast Cancer Prevention Partners, 2021). These numbers are astonishing and cause one to take a pause. Essentially one out of every three Black women who are stricken with breast cancer will not survive.

The intersection of being Black, a woman, and living in poverty predisposes Black women to health inequities, which is the embodiment of racism (Donnelly et al., 2020). You can often see health inequities manifest as ineffective patient-provider communication. Patient-provider communication, which includes multiple aspects of communication such as verbal and nonverbal interactions between patients and providers, are vital provisions of safe and high-quality healthcare. However, research illustrates that Black patients are more likely to experience inadequate communication when interacting with their providers. Janice's story throughout illustrates this inadequacy in regard to her treatment for breast cancer.

I applaud Janice for her honesty, candidness, and vulnerability. Janice's experience with breast cancer was like the rising phoenix. Although she endured a lot during her experience with cancer—grief, the loss of a romantic relationship, the loss of hair, new scars, body changes, and a health provider displaying blatant microaggressions—she reemerged a survivor. Although she emerged as only a fraction of the person she was, she developed new parts that were transformational. You know why? Because she's a warrior! That same warrior lives within you. Allow it to happen for you, not to you. Janice is a great example and embodiment of that statement.

A WAR OF THE WOMB

A Warrior Named Ayodele:
Her Battle with Uterine Fibroids

Advocate for yourself. Ask questions.
—Ayodele

Uterine fibroids disproportionately impact Black women (Stewart, 2013). Black women are three times more likely to develop uterine fibroids compared to White women (Grey, 2020). Further, Black women are more likely to develop uterine fibroid symptoms such as pain during sex, severe pelvic pain, long and heavy menstrual cycles, and anemia (Grey, 2020).

Ayodele, a 45-year-old Black woman experienced uterine fibroids, which led to a hysterectomy. Let's learn from this warrior about how uterine fibroids impacted her life.

Her Definition

Uterine fibroids are a cyst, a tumor, or a module. They can be as small as a pin but as large as a watermelon. They also cause severe pain and bleeding.

According to the Centers for Disease Control and Prevention (2021), uterine fibroids, the most common noncancerous tumors, are tissues and muscle cells that grow around or in the wall of the uterus.

Her Experience

I found out I had uterine fibroids about 20 years ago when I was pregnant with my oldest child. I experienced heavy bleeding and severe pain before starting my menstrual cycle. I was in pain all the time. The pain and bleeding got worse after I had her, although I had a cesarean delivery. I remember going to the bathroom at my new place of employment, using a tampon, and all of the blood splattering everywhere. It was all over the walls of the stall. I was like, *Oh shit, oh shit, oh shit, oh shit.* I was praying that no one would come in. I was thinking, *Please don't let anyone come in.* I was trying to wipe all of the blood off of the floor and walls of the stall. The first 2 days of my menstrual cycle were the worst. I would use a super tampon, sometimes two of them, and a super long pad. It felt like a damn dildo in your pants all day.

When I first experienced the pain and bleeding, I did not think anything was wrong. My mother told me that all of the women in her family experienced that. My mother had eight or nine sisters. It was just something that they dealt with until they had a hysterectomy. You know, strong Black women doing their stuff. So I said, "Well, I guess that's the road I have to go down eventually."

Her Well-Being

Uterine fibroids made me tolerate pain better. You learn to deal with stuff better because although you are experiencing pain, you have to work. So, hey, if I have to put in two tampons, that's what I am going to do. The heavy bleeding did cause me to be severely anemic; even though I've since had a hysterectomy, I'm still severely anemic.

After surgery, my emotional and mental health was impacted because they told me that the uterine fibroids were worse than expected. They had to remove an ovary and a fallopian tube. I remember breaking down. I was an emotional wreck.

Oh, and in regard to my physical health, I've always been a big girl. However, I've always been one to exercise. No matter what, I've always exercised. However, because of extreme blood loss every month due to my menstrual cycles, I became anemic and exhausted. I wasn't able to be as active as I wanted to be. I thought my midsection was super fat, but it was the fibroids. They were the size of grapefruits and made my abdominal area look bigger than it was.

I am constantly reminded of when the blood splattered all over the stall walls. After that experience, I went to the doctor. I will also always remember the extreme cramping that I experienced as a child. I was like, "What the hell?" Oh, and the pain. I would compare it to labor pains and contractions. I didn't realize that until I had my child. I also remember bleeding through my clothes a couple of times; I would bleed so much that the blood would leak through the tampon.

Her Support System

Everyone's advice in my support system was "Leave her alone, she's cramping," or "Leave her alone, her stomach hurts." When you're married or dating, I don't think your spouses or boyfriends or anyone know how to help. I don't want to say they don't care. But they don't know. I remember my husband saying, "P-M-S-ing again?" I genuinely don't think anybody who hasn't experienced uterine fibroids knows what to do or say. My mother knew what I was going through because she went through it. She would tell me to take Tylenol, get a heating pad, and that's about it. You have to keep on moving. I never called in sick to work. I had to pay rent.

I think my support system could have been improved if my husband would have said, "Okay, I know you're cramping and in pain; maybe take the day off?" Maybe? Instead, though, he said, "You're going to work, right?" That may have been more helpful. Now that I think about it, I would've had to miss work every month, and that wasn't an option. I had bills.

Her Intersection of Healthcare

I think my healthcare providers could have explained the information more. I didn't know anything about uterine fibroids until after I had my hysterectomy. I think they could have explained uterine fibroids more besides just saying it's a Black woman's thing. I think they could have provided more education. For instance, they could have described the symptoms, what causes uterine fibroids, and side effects. All I knew was that Black women get it, all my aunts had it, and it might require a hysterectomy. You bleed a lot, you cramp a lot, and you're cold because of anemia. That's it.

In the healthcare system, they do not provide detailed information. My healthcare providers didn't tell me I had endometriosis, how bad my uterus was, or that they would remove my fallopian tube or uterus. I also didn't know how my body and hormones would react after the surgery. They didn't explain any of that. Later, I learned there were other options to try before having a complete hysterectomy, and supposedly, Black women get hysterectomies faster than anyone else in the healthcare system. It bothered me after the fact because I wanted another child.

My experiences have taught me ask questions and advocate for myself. If something doesn't feel right, after about 10 days, I go to the doctor. If they aren't telling me what I want to hear, I ask more questions and insist on getting blood work.

Her Healing

I am still coping with uterine fibroids. I had my hysterectomy about 6 years ago. After the surgery, I am more hormonal. My hormones go haywire every other month, and I have to go to the doctor. I still experience some cramping although my uterus is gone because I still have one ovary and one fallopian tube. I don't have the heavy bleeding and hard pain anymore. I also get severely swollen and painful breasts. My milk ducts become full every two to three months. I didn't know this was going to happen. About five months after the hysterectomy, I thought I had breast cancer due to the pain and swollenness. I had a mammogram, and everything was fine. They told me it was just something I would have to experience.

However, if I had to do it over again, I would because I don't have to worry about carrying all that stuff around. I always had to ensure that I had tampons and pads. I kept them in the car. I kept them in all my purses. I kept them in my husband's car. I had to make sure that I was always prepared.

Moreover, my stomach went down, and I could fit into my pants. I like the fact that I don't bleed, so that's a huge accomplishment right there. However, I am still anemic and have to have iron infusions. My energy level is a lot better though, even if I'm still anemic.

Thinking about the past, if I could share a piece of advice with my younger self, I would ask questions. I would tell women to ask questions and don't let them tell you immediately that you have to get a hysterectomy. Research your options. When I think about my experience with uterine fibroids and reflect upon where I am now, I wish I had known more about uterine fibroids. During the period of slavery, Black women were strong. We need to remain strong; we can't be weak, tearful, or show emotions; we just always have to keep going.

As I reflect upon Ayodele's words, I am reminded of how the intersection of race, class, and gender impacts health outcomes for Black women. Although we do not conclusively know the risk factors for developing uterine fibroids, we know that health disparities are associated with it. We do know that Black women are more likely to develop uterine fibroids, are more likely to have severe symptoms, are more likely to wait to seek medical treatment, and are more likely to experience invasive procedures. And, we do know that Black women suffer in silence.

It is essential to understand the amount of suffering that Ayodele had to endure. Not only was she wearing one to two tampons and a pad, but she was also waking up every day and going to work. Too often, we become the strong Black woman, pushing and pushing while minimizing our pain until we can't push anymore. Many women think that their pain is normal.

When something doesn't feel right, understand that you don't have to be the strong Black woman and push through; go to the doctor if you can. On average, Black women seek medical treatment after 4.5 years of experiencing uterine fibroid symptoms, while White women seek medical treatment after 3.3 years of experiencing uterine fibroid symptoms (Grey, 2020). Early diagnosis and treatment are essential to improve health outcomes.

However, please note, when you go seek medical attention, ask questions. Despite alternatives that are minimally invasive procedures, Black women are two times more likely to get a hysterectomy than White women (Mostafavi, 2020). It is crucial to ask healthcare providers questions and do your research before agreeing to medical procedures. We must advocate for ourselves. You can do it. You are a warrior!

A Warrior Named Leah:
Her Battle with Polycystic Ovary Syndrome

Fight for your body until you find results that satisfy you.
—Leah

Polycystic ovary syndrome (PCOS), also known as polycystic ovarian syndrome, is a set of symptoms related to a reproductive hormonal imbalance (National Institute of Child Health and Human Development, 2017; Office on Women's Health, 2019a). PCOS occurs when a woman's adrenal glands or ovaries produce more male hormones than normal. Black women (8%) are more likely than White women (4.8%) to experience PCOS (Morgan, 2016). Common symptoms of PCOS include irregular menstrual periods; infertility; weight gain; pelvic pain; acne or oily skin; excess hair growth on the face, chest, stomach, or thighs; or patches of thickened skin. In this chapter, Leah, a 42-year-old married Black woman, discusses her experiences with PCOS.

Her Definition

I define PCOS as pain; that is what it is to me. Unfortunately, even though I was diagnosed with PCOS in 2009, my healthcare provider never told me I had it. I didn't find out until 2019.

PCOS is a reproductive hormonal disorder that may cause infrequent or prolonged menstrual cycles or excessive male hormones (Mayo Clinic, 2021). Moreover, the ovaries may fail to regularly release eggs or develop numerous small collections of fluid.

Her Experience

When my menstrual cycle began, it was very irregular. Once every 3 years, I would have a period, then maybe once a year, then once every 6 months. It wasn't until about 2 years ago that my cycle became regular—about every 45 days.

I was angry when I found out I was diagnosed with PCOS. The healthcare provider who diagnosed me never told me I had it. If I had known sooner, I could have sought help. It would have explained why I continued to experience miscarriages. There was a 10-year gap between my diagnosis and when I found out about my diagnosis.

Her Well-Being

PCOS impacted my mental health. I thought I was inferior because I was not able to have children. I did not understand why. However, later, I found out that it was due to PCOS. I was in shock. If I had known, I would have done what was needed to get better.

Additionally, if I had known, I would have advocated for healthcare providers to manage my pain better. My periods were so severe that I would vomit and have diarrhea. The pain would physically shock my body. Often, the healthcare providers made me feel as though my actions were intentionally causing the problem, like something was mentally wrong with me, rather than taking my concerns about pain and weight gain seriously. Every year, I would gain a couple pounds. Come to find out, it was due to my PCOS, not from my eating habits.

Learning about my diagnosis of PCOS calmed my spirit. Once I knew that I had PCOS, I understood why I was not able to have children. I understood why I continuously miscarried.

The time prior to learning I had PCOS took a toll on me. I made up so many issues in my mind about what was wrong with me, and you know, when your thoughts take over, you become emotional. It was horrible not knowing. However, once I found out, everything made sense, and I understood why my body was reacting the way it was.

Because of that, my physical health deteriorated. I struggled with a brain condition, pain, and weight gain caused by PCOS. Once I found out, everything improved because I had a better understanding of PCOS and how it was impacting my life.

When I think about my experience with PCOS, I think about my miscarriages. One of my most horrific PCOS experiences was when I had a tubular pregnancy. Unfortunately, I had to have emergency surgery. I was bleeding out. At that time, the healthcare providers knew I had PCOS, but I was not aware of my condition. I believe the surgeon thought the doctor who initially diagnosed me told me about the disease. There was probably a general belief that I already knew, which is why no one else said anything.

I compare the feelings of PCOS to severe cramping or being in labor. The vomiting and fever are like the flu. My body constantly fluctuated between being okay and not okay. Sometimes, I could barely walk because of the severe cramping or the shakes. I would be sick for 3 days. The first day was the worst; however, each day would get better.

Her Support System

No one in my support system knew that I had PCOS. When I found out, I did not tell anyone even though PCOS is major and massively affected my life. However, it wasn't deadly, so it didn't seem important enough to share.

Her Intersection of Healthcare

My experience in the healthcare system was horrible. I was miserable going to the hospital, getting shots, and not understanding why my cramping was severe. They wanted to put me on birth control, but it made me hemorrhage, and they could offer no other solution. They were basically like, "Well, I don't know what to tell you." Come to find out, I had PCOS, but no one told me.

It was not until I went in for my weight loss surgery that I learned about the PCOS. My provider tested from me head-to-toe for everything known to man. When my provider and I received the results, we discussed all the details to ensure that I was informed.

I should note that, for me, when navigating the healthcare system, it is not necessarily about being Black but rather about social class. Ultimately, my health insurance determined the type of healthcare that I received. If I had better health insurance, I probably would have been treated better and informed about my diagnosis. However, due to my class and insurance status, I was not.

Her Healing

Coping has become a way of life. I knew what to expect. I knew when I got a cold that it was the start of my menstrual cycle. Even though I knew what to expect, my body was still not handling my menstrual cycles well.

My biggest challenge was getting pregnant, and my biggest triumph was my little boy. After my weight loss surgery, my healthcare provider explained what was going on with my body. Losing weight and having my spine adjusted by a chiropractor helped me get pregnant. It all boiled down to knowing what was going on with my body and doing the things I needed to do to feel healthy and have a chance to get pregnant successfully.

My advice about POCS for other women is pretty straightforward. If you're experiencing consistent pain and having irregular or heavy menstrual cycles, it's okay to have your ovaries tested. I would not have had to struggle with all that pain all those years if I had known.

Let's take a look at Leah's story. Yet again, we see differences in health outcomes by race. One should note that differences in health outcomes by race are not solely due to genetics, cultural factors, or behaviors; instead, race-related health disparities are a physical manifestation of racism in this country (Donnelly et al., 2020).

While we do not know the causes of PCOS, poor patient-provider communication, possibly due to implicit bias, played a role in Leah's delay in finding out she had PCOS. Implicit bias is an essential contributor to race-related health disparities (Donnelly et al., 2020). Research links race-related implicit bias—negative subconscious beliefs—to explicit negative patient treatment, adverse health outcomes, and poor patient-provider treatment in Blacks. Withholding or even forgetting to provide pertinent medical information creates a conflict between healthcare providers' obligations to promote patient welfare and respect patient autonomy (AMA, 2021).

Imagine experiencing pain for 10 years and not knowing the cause. Imagine experiencing several miscarriages and not understanding why only to find out that you were diagnosed with PCOS and the previous healthcare provider failed to tell you. Tragic events like this have historically plagued Black women disproportionately and continue to do so. It's the harsh reality of a failed healthcare care system riddled with systemic racism.

Leah is a true definition of a warrior. I am inspired and encouraged by Leah. We must remember there is power in sharing your story and providing advice to other women. Imagine if another woman with PCOS had shared her story with Leah, Leah might have been able to seek help sooner. Remember, your story has the power to bless someone.

A Warrior Named Dioswal:
Her Battle with Polycystic Ovary Syndrome

Learn to be okay with letting things roll off your shoulders. Learn to not take everything to heart. And take the time to remind yourself: mind, body, and spirit.

—Dioswal

Due to the prevalence and varying symptoms of how PCOS impacts Black women, I wanted to continue the conversation. PCOS manifests in women's lives and affects them differently. So, let's hear from another amazing warrior about her journey living with PCOS. Dioswal is a 28-year-old Black and Asian American married woman. Let's learn from Dioswal how PCOS impacted her lived experience.

Her Definition

The way that I've come to understand PCOS is an imbalance in the hormones.

Her Experience

I was 8 or 9 years old when I experienced my first menstrual cycle. I noticed that I did not have a menstrual cycle every month. I asked my mom, and she mentioned that she and her sisters experienced the same thing. Therefore, I didn't think anything about it. When I was about 13 or 14 years old, I went to the doctor's office for my yearly exam. The doctor asked if my menstrual cycles were regular or routine. I replied, what's regular? She asked how many times per year did I have a menstrual cycle. I told them one to two times a year. That's when they diagnosed me with PCOS. They put me on birth control because they told me that I needed to have menstrual cycles due to my uterus not shedding its lining.

My experience with PCOS is rooted in my relationship with my dad. My dad had a negative view of women, especially Black women, which has impacted my perception of myself as a Black woman.

I was never a tiny kid in terms of being thin. My dad would say, "You should be smaller because you're half Asian." He would comment on how big my thighs and breasts were. I was self-conscious. My mom would also make me feel bad because whenever there was a momentous occasion, she would always say, oh, you can't get that because you're too big. She wasn't purposely trying to be mean.

During my senior prom, I went to Dillard's to find a prom dress. The store associate happened to be a Black woman. She could see how hurt and defeated I was after shopping. She said, "You have the body of a woman; you don't need to be shopping in that section." She did not make me feel bad. She spoke to me very lovingly. She was looking at my mom like don't make her feel bad about herself. It was at that moment that I realized that there's nothing wrong with me, you know? I just happened to have thickness in some places.

I didn't have an understanding of how PCOS could impact my life. The doctor did not say anything about infertility, hair growth, or weight gain. She only spoke about the irregular periods. She didn't treat it like a big deal; therefore, I didn't treat it like a big deal.

Her Well-Being

Due to PCOS, I struggle with my body image and Blackness. I struggle with what it means to be a Black woman. I'm still learning to reconcile it and accept what Blackness looks like for me. Additionally, weight gain has impacted my body image. It's been tough. I won't lie.

However, I've learned to become more in tune with my body and myself and step outside of religious dogma. I am learning how to be more intuitive.

I believe that being intuitive has propelled me into studying mental health counseling as a graduate student. Additionally, I started attending counseling. Through graduate school and counseling, I learned that I needed to change my diet and exercise. Once I started eating clean, I lost weight. By losing weight, my husband and I were able to conceive our daughter. She was my biggest blessing while on this journey.

Her Support System

To be honest, I didn't have support because my mom didn't know what it was. My dad didn't have an understanding of it either. However, once I got married, my husband became my support system. I remember looking at myself with a lot of disgust and discomfort because of how I looked. And to this day, you know, I've been married for a few years now and my husband hasn't looked at me any differently. He's taught me how to be comfortable in my own body and how to love myself, even at times when I don't feel like I deserved that. So, he's been a huge aspect of support.

Her Intersection of Healthcare

My experience with the healthcare system has been a hot mess. I mean, I cannot tell you the number of healthcare providers that I visited to shed more light on PCOS. I've literally just been passed over every time and been told, "You just need to lose weight," and I'm kinda like, "Well, no shit, Sherlock. I know that, you're not telling me anything different. But I'm actually having trouble trying to lose weight." I will never forget how a White nurse practitioner made me feel. I remember she was looking at my weight while reviewing my charts. She made a remark about my weight. I was like, "I know. I'm working on it." She had set up an appointment for me to a nutritionist. I saw the nutritionist and I was like, "This woman is talking to me like I'm stupid. I'm college educated. I'm working on my master's right now. Who the fuck do you think you're talking to?" I'm like, "I'm well aware of how all this works and you are not helping me at all." So, for me, a lot of the experience has been people talking down to me due to my weight.

Her Healing

I've been able to cope with having PCOS because I am blessed to have children. Many women who struggle with PCOS cannot have children. I'm very thankful. However, I still struggle with my body image and mental health. Some days are excellent, while some days are terrible, but counseling has been a tremendous help.

Looking back, I would educate myself about my reproductive system. While it's been an arduous journey, I am proud of myself for researching PCOS. I recently joined a PCOS support group. I enjoy engaging with women who also have PCOS.

Let's take a moment to reflect upon Dioswal's story. As we end the discussion, we must remember diseases and illnesses manifest differently in people's lives. In Dioswal's case, she was able to have children, whereas some women are unable to.

When you take a closer examination at Dioswal's story, it is clear that her healthcare providers did not inform her of the symptoms of PCOS until adulthood. Symptoms of PCOS often develop around the first menstrual cycle (Mayo Clinic, 2021). While it is not clear the direct correlation between PCOS and weight gain, women who experience PCOS often experience weight gain (Cleveland Clinic, 2021).

While weight gain cultivated body image problems, I applaud Dioswal learning positive ways to cope, specifically attending counseling and joining support groups. It is important to note that mental health counseling and support groups are beneficial when creating effective coping strategies.

Additionally, Dioswal struggled with her "Blackness." While the Black experience is not monolithic, we all want to feel a sense of belonging and connectedness. Fortunately, Dioswal has been working to reconcile those feelings.

Well, I am here to tell you, sis you belong. In everything you do, know that you belong. Understand that your Blackness is enough. Your Blackness was enough yesterday and will be enough tomorrow. And who you are and everything in you adds value to the culture. I am enamored with Dioswal because she did not allow her "Blackness" or body image defeat or define her. She has been doing the work to heal. She is a warrior who fought to find her healing!

A Warrior Named Heather:
Her Battle with Fertility

Fertility does not make me who I am, and it does not make any woman who she is.
—Heather

One of the most profound consequences of racism is its long-term, generational effects on health outcomes. Persistent and pervasive race-related health disparities in gynecologic healthcare continue to impact Black women's fertility. Black women are more likely than White women to experience fertility-related problems (Donnelly et al. 2020). We turn to the narrative of a warrior named Heather, a 41-year-old Black woman, to gain a better understanding of these issues. Here's Heather's story.

Her Definition

Fertility is the ability to have children—you know, being fertile.

As defined by Alexander et al (2017), fertility is the ability to produce offspring.

Her Experience

I miscarried when I was 21 years old, and then again at 37 years old. I've been pregnant twice and miscarried twice. I never got pregnant again. And here's the thing: I have never been on birth control.

Her Well-Being

Due to my fertility problems, I no longer want children. Further, I no longer want children due to how Black women are treated in America. It seems as though Black women get it harder than other races or ethnicities. Honestly, I think God was looking out for me. God knew what he was doing!

However, it is interesting to think about how my fertility has impacted my mental and emotional health, especially as a Black woman. When I miscarried, I was sad because I had to see other people with their children. It leaves you wondering at times. I guess it's just more challenging for me to have children. But now that I'm 40 years old, I think that ship has sailed. However, I often think about not being able to achieve having children, how hard it was to get pregnant, and the emptiness that I felt during my miscarriages.

Her Support System

Your support system is essential when you experience a miscarriage. During my first miscarriage, there was minimal support because was I was young. When I had my second miscarriage, the support was excellent. After the miscarriage, the father was very hands-on in making sure I was okay.

Her Intersection of Healthcare

I experienced my second miscarriage while visiting New Orleans, and the obstetrician was great. However, my first miscarriage was a different story. They sent me home very abruptly, like, "Oh, well, you lost a baby. Get over it." I think healthcare providers should be more hands-on, provide an adequate amount of time with you, and discuss the issues more. Minimally, they should at least have sympathy, be empathetic, and compassionate. Instead, I felt like they were pushing me out the door. Some doctors may be sympathetic, but when I was 21 years old, it was just like, "Well, you miscarried. Okay. Bye."

Her Healing

Despite all that I've experienced, I can cope with my fertility issues. It doesn't bother me anymore because growing up I never wanted kids. When I got older, I decided I wanted kids, but then I changed my mind again. I think it's too much responsibility.

The challenge of getting pregnant, trying to stay pregnant, losing the baby, and realizing I would never have a baby has been devastating. However, looking back, I would tell my younger self that it will happen when it happens. It is hurtful, and it will take time. I know it's rough, but for any other woman experiencing fertility issues, you will find your way through it. You don't always understand, but some things are inevitable, and you have to remain strong and take your time to get through them.

I can say that I am in a good space. I'm happy that I do not have a bunch of children, and it's just me. I do have a boyfriend, but without him, it would just be me, and I don't think that would be fair to my children.

Let's reflect upon Heather's story. By living in a race-conscious society, so often, Black women experience double jeopardy—that is, being Black and being a woman (racial and gender discrimination). As I reflect upon Heather's tale, I am reminded of how deeply racism impacts health outcomes for Black women. I am reminded that health disparities in gynecologic healthcare continue to impact Black women's fertility. I am reminded that Black women suffer in silence. I am reminded that Black women need support, and I am further reminded that too often Black women are dismissed in the healthcare system—a system that would easily use us for experiments, yet deny us adequate healthcare. For generations, we have been treated as less than human while the healthcare system has used our Black bodies for experimentation (Tuskegee Syphilis Experimentation).

Perinatal loss related to fertility-related problems creates a unique type of grief. It is a deeply profound experience one goes through that is not seen or noticed by the world. I am encouraged and empowered by Heather. It is important to understand Heather's feelings on a deeper level. If you decide to continue to try and get pregnant, that is okay. If you decide that you no longer want to try and get pregnant, it is okay. As Black women, we must realize that our story is ours and our decisions are ours and we should stand firm on what works for us.

Have you tried to get pregnant, yet every month Aunt Flo still comes? If so, you've probably cried more tears than you can count and felt more emotions than you can bear. What do you do? Infertility can sometimes feel as if you're in a desert—alone, thirsting with desire for children, and unsure of where the answers will come from. The unmet dreams of not having a child due to fertility-related problems can often lead us to feel empty, as if our goals are unachievable. Such despair leaves us to suffer in silence or carry a huge burden on our shoulders. Listen, you are a warrior! You are filled with purpose. You need to walk with authority and overflow in your abundance. There is nothing empty about you, sis.

A WAR OF BIRTH

A Warrior Named Asantewa:
Her Battle with Pregnancy and Childbirth

Pregnancy and childbirth were magical mysteries that I feel humbled, proud, and grateful to have experienced and witnessed through my own body.

—Asantewa

Compared to White women, Black women are more likely to experience maternal health complications during pregnancy and childbirth. Due to these maternal health complications, Black women are three to four times more likely to experience pregnancy- and childbirth-related deaths despite socioeconomic status and educational attainment (National Partnerships for Women and Families, 2018). Now a warrior named Asantewa shares her experience with pregnancy and childbirth. Asantewa is a 38-year-old married Black woman. Let's examine her story.

Her Definition

I would define pregnancy as carrying a child. Pregnancy is when your body is creating life. In regard to childbirth, that is when you are birthing a baby who is now ready to take on the world itself.

According to the National Institute of Child Health and Human Development (2017), pregnancy is defined as the period that a fetus develops within the womb of a woman.

Her Experience

My new African identity, African-centered ideology, and African-centered culture greatly influenced how I navigated my pregnancy and childbirth experience. It helped me to think about pregnancy and childbirth in a very positive way. Within African culture and spirituality, pregnancy and childbirth are considered rites of passage.

During that time, I recognized that I am a vessel who's bringing forth a baby, so I did what I needed to do to make it a joyous experience. I sat back and allowed my body and the universe to do what it was created to do.

I knew I was pregnant maybe a couple of hours before I took a pregnancy test. My husband and I had just eaten a big meal, and like 30 minutes later, I was still hungry; then, I wanted beer. I am not a beer drinker, so I knew something was going on.

My experience with pregnancy and childbirth was very pleasant. My husband and I were trying to get pregnant. I was very happy. The happiness carried through until maybe at about five or six months of pregnancy. After that, I started experiencing hormonal changes such as mood changes and strong food cravings. I'm always trying to be mindful and think that I'm in control, but I realized that oh, no, I'm not in control of these hormones. They were in control of me. My mood would just shift, and there wasn't anything that I could do about it. However, overall, it was pleasant.

In regard to childbirth, it was an interesting experience. I'm the youngest of seven, and I have four older sisters. We had all planned that they would be there, but my daughter came two weeks early. Thus, the people who were planning to be there—my best friend and my sisters—were not there. However, my husband, niece, and doula were.

I didn't feel much pain, and I know that sounds crazy. I remember letting out these big moans, but it was really like a big sigh. It wasn't like a cry of pain. I actually felt pain after, but the feeling during birth was euphoric. It was joyous.

I used mindfulness and African-centered spirituality to create a space that I felt was conducive to all the things I wanted. I had a natural birth and doula. I created a peaceful atmosphere and even made a music playlist. I had essential oils in the hospital room. I also had a big picture of my mom, who passed away a few years ago. This was significant because my mom was actually a midwife in her early years, and she played an integral role in all of my sister's birthing experiences, and I had always expected her to do that for me. Thus, I carried a sadness throughout my pregnancy and birthing process because I really wanted her to be here. However, her picture was a source of my strength.

Her Well-Being

Prior to pregnancy and childbirth, I had Superwoman Syndrome. I have always believed that I'm powerful and I'm strong, but I felt like I had a special power during the whole pregnancy. If I'm having an emotional day, I think about the fact that I was able to channel my emotions and control as much as I could. That makes me feel more empowered.

During my experience with pregnancy and childbirth, I felt connected to my spirituality. While I was pregnant, I was bearing witness to being a part of a vessel for something that doesn't make sense—it's only the spirit. Spirit and God, the unseen, the unknown, are all that can explain how birth happens; it's a real miracle. That grounded me in my spirituality, in a sense. I have even more faith in the unseen, in magic, and in mystery because of this experience.

Going back to being Superwoman, I think pregnancy created another layer of responsibility for me as it relates to my mental and emotional health. Black women are responsible for so much; mental and emotional labor, emotional intelligence, and emotional capacity all fall on us. However, it also taught me to really protect myself, so I protect my emotional and mental well-being now in ways that I never have before.

In regard to physical health, I'm motivated to maintain physical fitness. However, there are times that I feel tired, physically. Two days after childbirth, I felt like I got hit by a Mack truck. I could barely stand up. I tiptoed around the house. Physically, I didn't feel like I had any strength. They say that you use every muscle in the vaginal area. A couple months after I had her, I snapped back. It looked like I didn't have a baby at all. The weight came later because I wasn't as active. All the lying in bed, the recovery, plus eating more because now I'm breastfeeding, and now caring for this child means I'm using up energy a lot faster.

Thinking back about childbirth, my playlist comes to mind. I had a playlist of mostly India Arie songs. I used her most recent album, the one where she's meditating; it was like a whole meditation album pretty much, especially her song, "I Am Light." I had that one replaying during the birthing experience and before. That's one of my most vivid memories, of hearing that and really allowing, like I said earlier, myself to kind of transcend all the fear that I had in my head, all the anxiety that had built up.

My *blessing way* was another memorable moment. We call it a blessing way and not a baby shower. It's blessing the way for the baby and the mom. I came down to Atlanta, and my sisters were there. It was a great experience because I was showered with so much love—to the point where I could feel the baby moving as people shared their words of encouragement and wisdom.

I also remember my eight-bowl ceremony, which uses different spices of life that we taste. We use cayenne pepper for hot and critical times, lime for bitter times, and so on. Everybody gathered around and each person took a different element to talk about. One said, "Girl, you know you're going to have some bitter times with this baby." Whoever had honey talked about the sweetness, you know, of having a child and being a mother. We went through these eight different elements of life, or spices, and they're all foods. Coconut represents blessings. The water comes after the cayenne because it's supposed to cool you, and it represents the cool and level head that you have to have throughout motherhood. That was memorable. We also did a bead ceremony in which everybody would pick a bead out of a bowl, put the bead on a string, and talk about what that bead means. I had those beads actually in the hospital room when I gave birth because of all the energy that they put into them. They would choose different colors and say, for example, "I chose yellow because I want your child to shine bright like the sun."

Her Support System

I had a good community of people for my support system. All my sisters, even my father. In addition, I got my doula pretty early on. I don't remember exactly how far along I was, maybe about four or five months, and I had mentioned to a colleague, "Hey, do you know any Black women doulas?" I had always heard the benefits of having a doula. He recommended his wife, who was a doula. We started right away devising my birthing plan—my dream and vision—and I felt tremendously supported by her. With her support, I didn't feel like I was going through it alone. I had my husband and niece, but it was just us three in Ohio. I went from kind of feeling alone to feeling like I had a partner in this thing because my husband, even though he's my partner, doesn't know anything about being pregnant.

Having my doula and talking with other mothers was a crucial aspect of my support system. I was able to talk to my sisters, my aunts, and other women who had given birth. Being able to talk to them, and also to my best friend, you know, even though she hasn't had children, it was good to talk to her too because while the other women knew where I was going to, my friend knew where I was coming from.

Her Intersection of Healthcare

As a professor of Pan African Studies who understands Black people's history with the medical system and because of my own upbringing in an activist household, I have always mistrusted the medical system. I went into my pregnancy with a very healthy kind of mistrust. I did my research to make sure the healthcare providers were not leading me astray. I had a healthy dose of skepticism. I think my outlook caused me to be defensive and to feel like I had to be my own doctor. I interpreted their statements as them giving me recommendations or suggestions that I could take or leave.

My most memorable moment within the healthcare system during my pregnancy and childbirth was when I felt that my doctor caused me to have an early birth. It was actually 2 days after I had gotten an exam. She asked me if I wanted to check the position of the baby. I told her no because at that time, I was 4 weeks away from my due date. I had a discussion with my aunts—one of my aunts is a nurse and my other aunt is a doctor—and they both told me that at that stage don't have them check you because you're too far along. However, the doctor said something to make me agree. Previously, she had checked me and the baby was breeched—feet first instead of head first, so that's what we were checking and what we were concerned about. I said, "Yeah, we can check but you cannot go too far because you know, I'm listening to what my aunts told me." Long story short, she put her hand up there really hard and forcefully, to the point where I screamed. I think that she ruptured my sack because I went into labor 2 days later.

Her Healing

I coped by talking to other Black women who affirmed that what I was feeling and going through was normal. My biggest triumph during pregnancy and childbirth was that I was able to have a baby with no drugs even though the first contraction was just super intense. I felt it from my head to my toes. I was so proud of myself for being able to endure in spite of the pain. The turning point was when I just recalibrated and called on the spirit and wisdom of ancient African Black mamas who have been doing this since the beginning of time.

If I had to share advice with my younger self, I would say to trust your body. Be mindful. Be present to everything that you're going through. Don't wish it away, embrace it because actually all the feelings that you're having are preparation for when you actually give birth. What you feel during the pregnancy—the discomfort, the worry, the sickness, the pain, and the strain on your body—is preparing you for the actual birthing experience. Moreover, the birthing experience is preparing you to actually be a mother after the fact. All the things that you have to employ during pregnancy and childbirth are things that you'll have to continue to carry forward into motherhood.

My advice to other women is to trust themselves. I can't say that enough because we're taught not to trust ourselves. We're taught to trust the doctor, not ourselves, and that has gotten us into a lot of trouble. Sometimes, for example, we know we may feel a certain way, and then the doctor will discount or discredit us or not really give credence to the issues that we bring to their attention. Then, we start to believe the doctor instead of ourselves. Instead, continue to trust yourself. Your body knows. Listen to your body, and listen to your baby because that's something that's happening that's supernatural, that's outside of you. If you believe in God and you believe in spirit, if you believe in a higher being, then you have to believe that there's something that's happening that that has more wisdom than you or the doctor.

Let's reflect. One cannot examine pregnancy and childbirth among Black women without recognizing how living in a race-conscious society and the intersection of race, class, and gender have impacted health outcomes. When examining the healthcare system in regard to pregnancy and childbirth, one must note that 75% of Black women give birth in hospitals that serve predominantly Black populations (National Partnership for Women and Families, 2018). These predominantly Black-serving hospitals have worse health outcomes, such as pregnancy and childbirth-related complications, elective deliveries, and nonelective cesarean births. Further, there is a lack of effective patient-provider communication (Bergman & Connaughton, 2013). It should be noted that effective patient-provider communication significantly predicts trust among healthcare providers and Black women during pregnancy and childbirth. More specifically, research has shown that trust is related to satisfaction with care (Bergman & Connaughton, 2013).

Due to patient-provider communication being a concern, I applaud Asantewa for empowering herself and obtaining a doula. Doulas provide emotional, mental, physical, and educational support before, during, and after pregnancy and childbirth (Maternal Health Task Force, 2020). Further, research has demonstrated that Black women who utilize a doula are less likely to experience pregnancy- and childbirth-related deaths.

If you are trying to conceive or find yourself pregnant, I recommend seeking out the support of a doula. They will advocate for you when you can't advocate for yourself. They will motivate and support you when you feel alone. You can have a safe and enjoyable pregnancy. You can do it. You are a warrior!

A Warrior Named Kamesha:
Her Battle with Breastfeeding

Nourishing your baby through breastfeeding is one of the most important things you can do.

—Kamesha

Disparities exist in breastfeeding initiation and continuation (Li et al., 2019). Research reveals that Black women are less likely to intend, initiate, and continue to breastfeed than women in other racial groups (McKinney et al., 2016). Let's turn to a warrior named Kamesha to gain a better understanding of her experience breastfeeding. Kamesha is a 41-year-old married Black woman. Here is her story.

Her Definition

I define breastfeeding as nursing your child at your breast with your breast milk. It doesn't matter how often you do it.

According to the World Health Organization (2008), breastfeeding is defined as infants receiving breast milk, including milk expressed or from a wet nurse.

Her Experience

When I think about my experience with breastfeeding, race and class dynamics played a role. I grew up in a predominately Black, mostly lower-class neighborhood. As a result, I rarely saw anyone breastfeeding. Almost everyone that I knew used formula, although two of my cousins were breastfed well into their toddler years, and my family made jokes, calling them "breastfed babies." It was never perceived as a positive. Therefore, my perception of breastfeeding was impacted.

However, I was still determined to breastfeed. My experience with breastfeeding was challenging. When I had my daughter, I was able to immediately do skin-to-skin, and she latched on within the first hour. It was very painful because breastfeeding causes uterine contractions. I became discouraged and overwhelmed. Finally, I decided to call the lactation consultant. I was ringing the hospital bell every 30 minutes. I was asking all types of questions. Is it supposed to feel like this? Is this right? Is she latched on correctly? What's wrong? I remember one of the nurses walked into the room, grabbed my breast, and started squeezing it to demonstrate how to breastfeed. I thought, *Um, wait a minute, you just walked up to me and yanked my breast; hold on a second.*

Subsequently, I was discharged but ended back up in the hospital after delivery due to preeclampsia. During this time, they were trying to stabilize my condition; therefore, my doctor discouraged me from having my daughter visit. While in the hospital, I had to start breast pumping, which was earlier than most moms. I had to pump every hour. It was excruciating. My breast was so raw and tender. My nipples started to bleed. It got to the point where one of my nipples had a huge slice in it, almost as if it was going to fall off. I was pumping about 70% milk and 30% blood. The lactation consultant said it looked like strawberry milk.

Her Well-Being

Ultimately, I breastfed my daughter until she was 22 months old. A lot of the women, even the ones in my family, questioned why I was still breastfeeding. I was in it for the long haul because I realized that women in other countries breastfed until their child was 5 or 6 years old due to the nutritional benefits. In my experience breastfeeding, I received mixed feedback from Black women. They made comments such as, "You are going to spoil her." However, other Black women would say, "Oh, my gosh. That is amazing."

Breastfeeding in public was a challenge for me, especially, in the beginning. I'm a private person, but after a while you just stop caring about when or where you feed your baby. The baby has to eat. I got a couple of rude looks, but I would look back, real stank. I became hypersensitive because historically Black women's bodies are oversexualized. I made sure to equip myself with the Ohio laws regarding breastfeeding in public places in case someone tried to challenge me. If my drape fell, my husband was always there to pick it up.

Breastfeeding was like an out-of-body experience. I was able to nourish life. I felt empowered. God was giving me the ability to nourish and produce the antibodies my daughter needed. If she were sick or cranky, I would breastfeed to soothe her. When my daughter was 5 or 6 months old, she caught a stomach bug. She couldn't keep anything down. I called the nurse hotline. The nurse told me to breastfeed her, and she would be able to keep that down. I nursed her, and she did not vomit.

Breastfeeding taught me that I was resilient. Once I made my mind up, there's nothing I couldn't do, even when faced with adversities. It was a moment of empowerment.

Breastfeeding was also good for my health. One of the little known facts about breastfeeding is that you burn an abundance of calories by breastfeeding, so I lost a ton of weight. In addition, I was also conscious about what I was eating because it would affect my daughter. I remember one time I was eating onions. I quickly found out that when I ate onions and breastfed, she would have gas.

The last time I nursed my daughter, she was 22 months old. I remember the last night I nursed her; I thought that I wouldn't offer her any in the morning or the evening. As I nursed her, she fell asleep. I laid in her bed, then walked out of the room crying. Something came over me spiritually. The next day, I didn't offer it, and just like that, it was over.

Her Support System

While I was breastfeeding, my support system was essential. I attended breastfeeding support groups, but they were one-sided. If I went, I went, and if I didn't attend, no one would miss me. Moreover, I was the only person of color in the group. I remember looking around and naturally being very conscious of that. However, my good friend from childhood encouraged me. We would have virtual breastfeeding sessions. She would give me tons of advice. My husband was also helpful and made so many sacrifices. He would run all of the errands so I wouldn't have to take my daughter out of the house.

Her Intersection of Healthcare

The healthcare system offered me very little support regarding my breastfeeding efforts. Had I not been determined, I would have stopped breastfeeding. I did not receive support unless I sought it out, attended a support group, scheduled an appointment, or called the lactation consultant. If I hadn't taken the initiative, I would not have gotten what I needed. Further, there weren't many, if any, conversations about breastfeeding at my daughter's pediatrician appointments.

The healthcare system should have lactation consultants who can come to your home and demonstrate different postures and methods and tools; if you don't have a specific item at home, they would be able to instruct you on other items you need to get.

I am thankful that I met one nurse who volunteered to come to my home, unpaid, to help me with breastfeeding. She had three children and experienced several breastfeeding complications. Therefore, she was willing to do whatever she could to help moms.

Her Healing

Breastfeeding was challenging because often I had to seek out information and support on my own. My biggest challenge was not having any support from health practitioners. If it weren't for my friend, who is also a Black woman, I'm not sure what I would have done.

Thinking back, if I had to give my younger self advice about breastfeeding, I would still breastfeed. It is critically important for our babies. If you can breastfeed—I know some moms can't—but if you can, do what you can for your baby. Breastfeed when you can, as long as you can. I'm very skeptical about what's in the formula.

I would advise women to seek out encouragement from other Black women who breastfed. It is natural to nurse your baby. You have to learn as you go. Like most parts of being a parent, you can never be sure if you're doing it right. I'm surprised that I was.

Now let's reflect upon Kamesha's story about breastfeeding. Breastfeeding is essential to reduce unfavorable pregnancy outcomes, specifically infant morbidity and mortality (Evans et al., 2021). Infants who were breastfed have significant reductions in sudden infant death syndrome and infections such as ear, gastrointestinal, and respiratory infections.

Although breastfeeding benefits are clear, unfortunately Black women do not initiate and continue breastfeeding for long periods. This is often due to (a) Black women's labor participation, (b) Black women's bodies historically being oversexualized, and (c) healthcare system challenges (Echols, 2019).

In regard to Black women's labor participation, about 80% of Black women are the primary providers of their households (Spates et al., 2020). Black women often occupy jobs that do not offer economic stability, flexibility, and paid family leave (American Civil Liberties Union, 2021). Therefore, after birth, many Black women experience financial stressors that force them to return to work, oftentimes earlier than other races.

Historically Black women's bodies have been dehumanized and oversexualized, which has impacted Black women's breastfeeding choices (American Civil Liberties Union, 2021). During slavery, Black women were historically forced to wet nurse for White families, which has created a complex, traumatic ideology around breastfeeding.

Finally, as you can see in Kamesha's story, the healthcare system poses tons of challenges for Black mothers trying to breastfeed. Although some resources are available, there is often a lack of support by the healthcare system.

I applaud Kamesha because, although faced with many challenges, she found resources and support and was able to breastfeed. Kamesha is the epitome of perseverance. As challenging as it may seem, ladies, know that you can do it when you put your mind to something. Even if it looks like you are not getting the support you need, know that there is a warrior deep inside of you that will push through any adversity. If you ever have to bet on someone, make sure you bet on yourself because you got this!

A WAR OF LOSS

A Warrior Named Antonique:
Her Battle with Miscarriage

My story is one of hope, healing, and a reminder of God's promise of beauty for ashes.
—Antonique

Research has determined that Black women are two times more likely than White women to experience an increased risk of miscarriage, specifically in gestational weeks 10–20 (Mukherjee et al., 2013). In this chapter, a warrior named Antonique narrates her experience with miscarriage. She is a 37-year-old, married Black woman. Let's dive in.

Her Definition

I define miscarriage as a loss of pregnancy.

According to the Centers for Disease Control and Prevention (2020c), miscarriage refers to the loss of a baby before the 20th week of pregnancy.

Her Experience

My culture, West Indian, has influenced how I navigate the world in terms of having miscarriages. I have had four miscarriages. My last miscarriage was in July of 2017. That miscarriage was the most impactful of the ones I've suffered. In that pregnancy, I knew the gender and even named her. I felt like, "Okay, this is it. This is finally happening," after three times before. Each miscarriage leaves you feeling defeated. You grieve more with each one. More questions pop up, like, "Am I ever going to be a mom?" or "What's wrong with me?"

I had so many questions. I grieved hard for the baby. I was on bed rest, doing all the things I was supposed to do. I went in for a test, and there was no heartbeat. It was literally like carrying death around inside of you. The trauma from that pregnancy affected my pregnancy a year later.

Her Well-Being

When I experienced my miscarriages, I felt like I was losing my mind. I remember certain days, such as Mother's Day, that would trigger me. I noticed that my energy was down and I was slowly developing depression.

I was struggling. However, I was introduced to an organization called A Little Piece of My Heart, which provides support and awareness to all who have experienced a miscarriage. The organization allowed us to share our stories, which was beneficial because most women won't share their stories due to shame and guilt. As a Black woman, it made me more aware of other Black women going through the same thing and how we needed to advocate for ourselves and each other due to the disparities in fetal health.

Additionally, I also created an inspirational playlist to help me cope. The music changed the atmosphere. Spiritually, journaling also helped. When I started the healing process, I would cry all the time. I would go to the cemetery where my daughter was buried, sit on the bench, journal, and listen to my playlist. I felt like God was speaking to me and letting me know that life will be okay. My heart tells me that God was renewing and strengthening my faith. That was after surrendering the pain over to God.

Her Support System

My support system is interesting. I have a blended family, and my husband's children were supposed to come to town. On the day that I experienced my miscarriage, my husband went to New York to pick up his children and left me. I needed him to stay, and I thought it was insensitive that he would bring the children back. I needed time to grieve the loss of my child. I just needed some time. However, my grandmother was there, and she took care of me. He felt like I would be okay because she was there, but the truth is I needed him in those moments.

I also found a support system by looking up different hashtags that deal with miscarriage. I found myself reaching out to people or silently following them on social media to look at their inspirational quotes.

Her Intersection of Healthcare

The healthcare system shaped my experience with miscarriage because I realized that I had to advocate for myself. When the healthcare providers walked into the hospital room, they looked at my kinky curly hair, heard my West Indian accent, and they talked to me rudely. I found myself having to be assertive.

Her Healing

I realized how strong I am, although I am still coping. I feel immense strength and tenacity. However, I had challenges. My biggest challenge was my support system. My family was miles away in the Bahamas. I was alone. In addition, all of my friends had moved away. However, now I can say that my most significant triumph is talking about my baby without crying. I have healed in some small way, shape, or form. I also like the fact that I am having this conversation now because people don't normally talk about miscarriages in my culture.

My turning point in my life when experiencing my miscarriages came at that moment when I felt like enough is enough. I knew I had to change. I was about to check myself into a mental hospital because I was starting to have suicidal ideation. I realized it was overwhelming my life and making me insane. I was going crazy. I had to get a hold of myself. It was at that moment that I decided that I cannot go down like this. I can't do this.

If I had to give my younger self some advice, I would tell myself to always remember that you're stronger than you ever know. Don't be afraid to tell your story because it's not only empowering and healing for you but for others. I would tell women to build a support system because that's important. Tell your story. Write it down. Talk about it.

As I reflect upon Antonique's interview, I reflect upon how Black women, yet again, experience another health disparity. I reflect upon how even when you control for age, alcohol use, and other factors, Black women still experience more miscarriages than White women. I reflect upon how research details how the differences in miscarriage rates are linked to race (Mukherjee et al., 2013).

The loss of an infant via miscarriage creates a unique type of grief. Black women experience stressors related to suicidal thoughts, self-blame, shock, and sleep disturbance (Boyden et al., 2014). It is an experience that the woman often may experience alone.

Antonique empowers me. The thought of experiencing several miscarriages is devastating. However, sometimes after the storm a rainbow comes. Antonique was able to give birth to an amazing rainbow baby.

What do you do when it feels like your world is turned upside down? What do you do when everything you hoped and dreamed for seems to be taken away from you? What do you do when all the ideas you had are no more? You fight. You continue to choose yourself every day. You continue being that warrior you were called to be!

A Warrior Named Skye:
Her Battle with Infant Mortality

God said that He needed him more than I did. So there's nothing I could do. I got an angel on my shoulder.

—Skye

Despite leading the world in healthcare advances for newborns, there are stark disparities in infant mortality rates in the United States. Black infants are approximately 2.3 times more likely to die than White infants (Centers for Disease Control and Prevention, 2019). Data from Centers for Disease Control and Prevention revealed that infant mortality rates were 10.75 per 1,000 live births for Blacks compared to 4.63 per 1,000 live births for Whites in 2018 (Ely and Driscoll, 2020). Let's turn to a warrior named Skye to gain a better understanding of her experience with infant mortality. Skye is a 44-year-old Black woman.

Her Definition

I would define infant mortality as an infant passing away from issues that may be able to be treated.

Infant mortality is defined as the death of an infant prior to the age of one (Centers for Disease Control and Prevention, 2020c).

Her Experience

When I was 6 months pregnant, I was lifting heavy groceries. A couple hours after lifting the groceries, my mucus plug came out. I called my sister and informed her that I was cramping, and she told me to contact my healthcare provider. When I called my healthcare provider, they told me to go to the hospital. Once I got to the hospital and was examined, they told me I was in active labor and three centimeters dilated.

My healthcare providers gave me steroid shots to develop my baby's lungs since I was going into preterm labor. After receiving the steroid shots, they told me that I would be in the hospital until the baby came. They kept me in a position where my feet were higher than my head to ensure that the baby would not come. I went to the hospital on October 27, 2002, and I gave birth on Saturday, November 2, 2002, at 9:39 p.m.

When my son Shaun was born, I was able to hear him cry. I take great pleasure in the fact that I got to hear him cry, at least that one time, because that's the only time that I heard him cry. They immediately put him on a respirator, and then he remained in the hospital for the next 12 weeks.

Two weeks after my son was born, he contracted a bacterial infection called pseudomonas. Pseudomonas is detrimental to children. Out of every 10 children who are diagnosed, only three survive because pseudomonas is a gram-negative bacterial infection; therefore, it can be antibiotic-resistant.

Due to pseudomonas, his blood pressure would shoot really high, then really low. Therefore, he experienced brain trauma. On one side of his brain, he experienced Level 3 brain trauma, and on the other side, he experienced Level 4 brain trauma. The doctor warned us that there was a good chance that Shaun would be a vegetable. They told us that he would also be on a respirator his entire life.

Although Shaun beat pseudomonas, it was too much for his body. He was in critical condition. Therefore, the hospital asked his dad and I if we wanted to do comfort care. We said no, we would like to do everything to sustain our child's life. They proceeded to tell us that the hospital board, called the ethics committee, was going to meet and vote on whether Shaun should receive comfort care. Ultimately, the hospital voted against our wishes to start Shaun's comfort care on a Monday.

One of Shaun's nurses informed us that we could have him transferred to a different hospital. However, Shaun passed away on January 25 at 9:34 pm before we were able to initiate the transfer and prior to start of comfort care.

I remember the day like it was yesterday. Shaun's dad and I were arguing all day long. Finally, I left and went to the hospital because Shaun wasn't doing well due to his medication. The medicine caused his blood levels to be too acidic. When I got to the hospital, his heart rate continued to drop. The nurse informed me that she thought the time was coming. She let me know that none of the babies died alone. She mentioned how they were held when they passed away. After we spoke, she turned the ventilator's alarms to prevent them from continuously beeping due to his low stats. I held him for about an hour.

Afterward, I left to go pick up his dad to come and spend time with him. I also picked up my mother. When we got to the hospital, my mother told us to go see him, and she would be up after she parked the car. When we got on the neonatal unit, we washed our hands, and I felt something go through me. That's how I know the exact time he passed away because I felt him. However, I didn't know what was going on at the time.

Once we get on the unit, the nurse said, "Sorry for your loss." I screamed, "No, no, no, no, no!" They handed me Shaun, and I held him until his dad grabbed him. I took one of his blankets, smelled his scent, and fell to the ground. I couldn't believe my baby was gone. They sent a chaplain and psychiatrist to assist. When my mother got upstairs, she rubbed my back and got me off the floor. We sat there for about two hours while I said goodbye to him.

Her Well-Being

I was angry because all these crackheads can have healthy babies. I was struggling mentally and emotionally. It's hard to deal with. However, I realized that everyone has a different plight and cross to bear. If it doesn't break you, it will make you stronger.

I believe that Shaun walks with me and protects me. Shaun is an angel. He is no longer suffering or in pain. He wasn't going to live a regular life; he wouldn't have been able to crawl, laugh, play, or go on walks.

When Shaun was in the hospital, the staff gave me a poem that helped me put everything into perspective. I included it in his obituary. This is the poem:

A Place Where Children Live

What kind of place would heaven be with all its streets of gold,
if all the souls, that dwell up there like yours and mine were old?
How strange would heaven's music sound when harps begin to ring,
if children were not gathered round to help the angels sing.
The children that God sends to us are only just a loan,
He knows we need their sunshine to make the house a home.
We need the inspiration of a baby's blessed smile,
He doesn't say they've come to stay, just lends them for a while.
Sometimes it takes them years to do the work for which they come.
Sometimes in just a month or two. Our Father calls them home.
I like to think some souls up there bear not one sinful scar.
I love to think of heaven as a place where children are.

I feel as though God needed Shaun more. Thinking of him now, Shaun would be 19 years old this year. I often wonder what type of man he would be. I wonder about all of his milestones. It's good to know that I have an angel on my shoulder. Losing Shaun was like having my breath taken away because he was a part of me. Although I was only pregnant for 6 months, I got to feel him grow and develop.

Her Support System

I had a great support system. My family was there every step along the way, and they're still here today. I wasn't alone. They allowed me to talk and express myself. It makes it easier to go through tragic events without feeling judged. However, I do think that I should have gone to grief counseling.

Her Intersection of HealthCare

When I experienced Shaun's loss, one of my memorable moments in the healthcare system was when the doctor who performed the autopsy spoke with me. He was very friendly and answered all of my questions. I was very blessed that the doctors and nurses were nice.

Her Healing

I am able to cope by being able to talk about him and express my feelings. That's my biggest triumph, being able to keep his memory alive. Even though he passed away, he is still alive in my heart. I may not have gotten to see him grow and develop the way that I wanted to, but he gets to see me grow and develop. Sometimes that's how I look at it.

One of the hardest things was using the money that I had been saving to buy his baby stuff for a funeral. That was not my plan. However, my biggest challenge when dealing with his death was the amount of time it took me to get pregnant again. It took so long that I got to the point where I was okay with not having children. Ultimately, I had a daughter.

Looking back, if I had to give my younger self advice, I would say be more in tune with your body. If I had known then that it was my mucus plug, I would have gone to the hospital immediately. Listen to your body.

A child is a blessing, but unfortunately, he was not my child to keep. If you lose your child, know that your child is an angel looking out for you the rest of your life, so you have an angel on your shoulder, on your head, and on your back with their wings wrapped around you. You are still loved.

Let's reflect upon Skye's story. One must note the importance of an infant mortality rate. Infant mortality rates are used to measure the health and well-being of a population (U.S. Department of Health and Human Services, 2015), and infant mortality rates allow countries to compare their overall health statuses. The United States ranked 33 out of 36 in infant mortality among countries that participate in the Organization for Economic Co-operation and Development (OECD), meaning that the United States has one of the highest infant mortality rates of any developed nation (OECD, 2018). It should be noted that some underdeveloped nations outperform the United States in infant survival, which implies that some underdeveloped countries have better infant mortality rates than Black women in America, even when the Black woman is educated and has a higher socioeconomic status. For instance, Black women with a graduate degree and higher income have worse infant mortality rates than White women with a high school diploma. This discrepancy is unacceptable.

You may wonder why this is so. Cumulative effects on mental health and exposure to stress due to individual, institutional, and structural racism impact infant morbidity and mortality rates. This exposure to stress is often from day-to day discrimination, microaggressions, and biases in the healthcare system from the lack of effective patient-provider communication and access to quality healthcare.

As I reflect upon Skye's interview, I acknowledge how strong she is. It takes a certain level of strength to survive what she had to experience. No parents should ever have to bury their child. I applaud Skye for sharing her story and keeping Shaun's memory alive.

If you have experienced the loss of a child, there are no words to describe the pain that you've had to endure. However, I just want to tell you that even in your darkest moments, there is a pinhole of light to help you get through. Know that you are not alone, and a tribe of women are ready and willing to support you. You are a warrior!

A WAR OF THE MIND

A Warrior Named Jamila:
Her Battle with Postpartum Depression

Rising from the ashes.
—Jamila

Black women are twice as likely to develop postpartum depression as White women (Howell, 2005). However, although Black women are more likely to develop postpartum depression, they are 57% less likely to seek professional mental health treatment (Sandoiu, 2020). This situation is problematic due to the fact that Black women are at increased risk of experiencing suicidal ideation. Jamila, a 29-year-old married Black woman, details her experiences with postpartum depression. Here's Jamila's story.

Her Definition

Postpartum depression is the feeling that you've been separated from everything that you once knew. You feel as though you have to start over again—you feel lost. It seems to be a common theme, but it manifests differently in each person.

Postpartum depression, often called the baby blues, refers to depressive symptoms after childbirth (Office on Women's Health, 2019b).

Her Experience

The first time I experienced postpartum depression was when I gave birth to my first child, who is now 5 years old; I was suicidal. I knew I needed help. I had experienced depression before on varying levels, and I used to self-harm when I was younger. I felt myself revisiting that place in my life, so I knew I had to get help for the sake of my health and the health of my child.

I received outside help, went to therapy, and learned my triggers. Postpartum depression may be a hormonal thing, but when you give birth, you are also learning a completely different side of yourself, which can be very stressful. I realized that I suffer from major depression but it is also triggered by postpartum depression.

I remember it being hard to get out of bed. I remember it being a season of difficulties. I knew I would never harm my child, but I felt like he would be better off without me. That's why therapy helped a lot. Getting therapy was the best decision I could have made because I no longer felt like my son didn't need me.

Her Well-Being

Experiencing postpartum depression as a Black woman has changed everything. Now that I'm on the other side of it, I have had another child and again experienced postpartum issues. However, though I was depressed with my second child, the differences between the two pregnancies and births were drastic. My second pregnancy taught me to desire to be in rhythm with the energy I possess and be fluid and connected. I learned to feel the energy and connectedness. Instead of feeling worthless and not being able to do anything for months, I could accomplish things like folding laundry in a half day. I still feel the cloud that comes, but now I know how to open the umbrella instead of getting soaked by the rain.

Oddly, having postpartum depression as a Black woman gives me the ability to connect with other women. If you're in that place, I promise there is something on the other side of it. I promise there is an entirely new life and version of yourself that you never thought existed, and it has the power to be whatever you want it to be.

I also feel like I wouldn't be able to convey that message if I hadn't experienced postpartum depression. It feels like rising from the ashes because everything you knew about yourself changes after you give birth. After the birth of my first child, I felt deep loss and grief. Now, after the birth of my second child, I see it as an opportunity to rebirth myself. It is a positive thing for me now.

Postpartum depression is something we need to talk about, and the spiritual side of coping is also something we need to discuss much more. I was much younger with my first child and still trying to figure out what I wanted out of life and who I wanted to be as a partner and a mother. With my second child, I already knew what I wanted. At that point, I was in the foundation-building stage of my life.

Spiritually, I had to learn a daily practice for survival due to the depression.

This practice carried me through to my second child and on to the present, so it has become part of my being. It's something I am and do all the time. I'm still practicing going to my shrines and altars every day, but the connection I feel is so much stronger now than it was before because I don't have a choice if I want to be here for my family. I have to be well. I have to be balanced and have a firm foundation.

Postpartum depression made me realize that I have to be in touch with my emotions. I have to move through everything I feel and not brush it to the side. I can no longer say I'm going to figure out things later or that I'm going to ignore my emotions and keep doing my day-to-day duties. When I ignore things or put them off, they accumulate. I have to think through things and pray about them. When the feelings and thoughts come, what do they mean? Is this a pattern in my life? Is it connected to a routine? Is the thought or feeling connected to a trigger? Is it related to anything, and if so, what? How do I find what it is, and how do I go through it? I can now go through this process.

I'm no longer frozen in time and unable to do anything. I can process my thoughts and feelings and understand I'm going to work through it to get to the other side of it all. It's hard work, and sometimes it's terrifying because you have to look at the parts of yourself you don't want to see. Working through things holds you accountable for your own mental and emotional health. You cannot point fingers at others; you only have control over yourself. I realized I would never get to the other side if I didn't hold myself accountable for changing the things I control. I now have control and no longer feel lost and overwhelmed.

Initially, the depression affected my physical health because I was self-harming. Beyond the self-harming, it affected my physical health due to the food I chose to eat, not being active, and staying in bed for days at a time. Our emotions are held in our muscular tissues. When you're pregnant, you are carrying and growing a life inside of you, and everything in your body changes. Everything inside of you shifts—your bones and organs—and in giving birth, even if you have a C-section, your entire body is affected. If you're not focused on healing properly, what you experience turns into trauma, and all of that trauma is held in our bodies and turns into physical pain.

When I consider women's various experiences related to postpartum depression, I think about myself, my mother, and my grandmother. As a woman, you are born with all the eggs you will have for your entire life. I was in my mother's body and my grandmother's body when they were born. All of the DNA passed down through the generations. All of the information contained in those eggs stays with us.

Even though I gave birth to two boys and the passing down of information is a little different, they still lived in me from my birth. They are from me, and they get all of the experiences from me because it is encoded into their DNA from being part of my eggs. It makes me think of my legacy and what I pass on spiritually and physically. I think about the things that I touch and my environment, which also gets passed on to my kids. I think about my characteristics and how I deal with situations and mental illness because it runs in my family. I do not particularly appreciate saying it runs in my family, but generational trauma means generational healing needs to occur.

Carrying and birthing a child ties together everything I just mentioned—from the spiritual realm to the physical realm and to all of the paused things while you are creating and growing this life inside of you. You have to consider what happens after they're born.

The feelings I had with postpartum depression are hard to compare to anything else, but let me try for a second. In an episode of a show on Amazon Prime, Anne Hathaway played a character who had these dramatic highs and lows in her personality. It was theatrical in how it was filmed and put on, but it resonated with me because I was in theater in high school. She had scenes where she would have a bright smile, sparkly clothes, beautiful hairdo, and a wonderful life. Then there would be a sudden change on the set. The lights would go dark, and she'd drop her shoulders, lie down in the bed, and say she cannot get up. The switches were very prevalent when she was on an impromptu date and her mood swings were too low; her date was like, "What's going on? Do you not like me?"

That episode showed how it feels being a Black woman with postpartum depression. I'm generally a bright and happy person, but then the switch happens, and I have no energy, can't get out of bed, and am prone to tears. Previously, I had feelings of worthlessness, as if I was buried under everything. I felt like there was no point in making any contributions in life because I couldn't do so the way I wanted. I would be tired and had no desire to run around the house, so I would lie in bed, binge-watch TV, and play games on my iPad.

Her Support System

When you have depressive feelings and thoughts, it's essential to have a strong support system. During my second pregnancy, my husband (it was his first child) was amazing. He instinctively knew how to take care of me during the ups and downs of postpartum depression. He even took time off from work, which was a blessing because I know not all men can do that.

I also had my mom, my doula, and her best friend, who's a second mom to me. My sisters and grandma cooked food, and other people dropped off food for me. The community aspect of support is so critical. I had people checking in on me and bringing me food and making sure to take my eldest son to and from our relatives and other places he needed to be. I felt very taken care of, which helped alleviate the depression. I was extremely depressed during my pregnancies, so giving birth was a relief. I felt so badly for my husband because I was the meanest, worst version of myself that he could have ever experienced. Not only was I pregnant, it was also our first year living together, so it had its challenges. I knew the second time around, once my hormones leveled out a little bit, I would be okay. The second time around, I had my spiritual foundation. I told myself to continuously put huge offerings to the ancestors and spirit and acknowledge and be thankful that we made it through. I gave thanks to the spirit and the ancestors that we're still together as a family and that I'm safe and the baby's safe because I had complications on top of the depression. The light at the end of the tunnel was knowing that because I learned how to cope, despite the postpartum depression, we would all be okay.

One of the most beneficial things for me after I gave birth was that everyone allowed me space to heal. I had family members who brought food. My grandmother, God bless her, was a tremendous asset. I miss her so much. My mother-in-law, who lives in California, always called to check on me and to talk. I had an outstanding balance between talking, having visitors, and having my space. I really cannot think of anything that could have been better because everyone was so wonderful.

Her Intersection of Healthcare

In regard to how the healthcare system shaped my experience with postpartum depression, for both pregnancies, I had a team of midwives and delivered at the hospital because I could not afford an at-home birth, and home births are not covered by my insurance.

The healthcare system in the United States is not set up for the well-being of Black women. I have watched documentaries about our healthcare system, read books, and more. I wanted a natural birth and to make sure that I had a team that supported me. When I first got pregnant, I had no idea what all this was going to look like because I had never been pregnant before. I had a trusted team for the birth of my son, but I didn't feel connected to my primary care physician. When I started feeling depressed, I didn't know I could go back to my midwife team. I went to my primary care physician and she sent me to a young, white therapist with whom I had no connection. It was really hard for me to find help the first time around. I had to do a lot of research to find a therapist who I could connect to and trust with my story.

I'm privileged, and I understand that I'm privileged to have learned tools to be able to advocate for myself in that way. Unfortunately, not all women know how to do that. As a Black woman, you have to know how to seek things for yourself because it's not going to be handed to you. It's not going to be given to you. On top of that, you have to fight for what you deserve and be the best advocate you can for yourself.

The second time around, I knew better. I knew I needed to have therapy set up for myself before I gave birth. Despite refusing it my first pregnancy, I opted for antidepressants with my second pregnancy. In retrospect, I wish I would have just taken them the first time because they really made a difference. I chose to stick with one midwife for all my appointments, even when I had to drive out of town to see her, whereas I had a team of midwives for my first pregnancy. I drove to Hudson, Ohio, for every appointment because the midwife knew me and my history, and I trusted her. I refused to speak with anyone else.

Having postpartum depression taught me to advocate for myself in the healthcare system. It sucks, but it's what you have to do. Searching for a pediatrician and help with postpartum depression 3–4 days after giving birth is such a vulnerable time. It makes you not want to speak to anyone, not leave the house, and not want to deal with anything else. Because I needed mental health therapy, it was even more critical for me to have a pediatrician that I trusted because I was in my most vulnerable condition, and if I said the wrong thing to the wrong person, I would have had Child Services at my door. It forced me to be extra careful with who I kept around me and where I sought help because I did not want to cause a snowball effect. I had to learn how to advocate for myself in a way that would not draw negative attention but rather show that I was in complete control of my situation.

I remember taking my second son to the pediatrician one time and having to fill out a first-time visitor form. The questions seemed much different than what I saw with my first son. Postpartum depression was more acceptable by the time I had my second son, but I don't remember them asking me all these questions with my first child. The questions were triggering. I had to stop and think through things thoroughly before answering and make sure I was not speaking from a place of depressed thoughts. Is this how I'm feeling right now or are these feelings old? Are these feelings from a pattern, a trigger? Am I taking care of myself? I have to run through all those questions any time I fill out one of those questionnaires.

Add to all of that the fact that Ohio is *country*, and you can imagine how I felt as I sat in the doctor's office—the only Black person there. I know people reading this may question whether Ohio's country, but it really is! We have a few nice cities, but for the most part, it's country. I'm in the office, answering these triggering questions and trying to calm myself down, manage my emotions, and prepare myself for the conversation with the doctor. In my mind, I represent Black women everywhere because not everyone advocates for us.

The doctor in Hudson was much better than the one I had in Akron. The one in Akron was rude, and none of the staff there cared about me. Being in

Hudson was stressful, though. Every time I went there, I had to consider how I spoke to people because I wasn't sure how much interaction they had had with Black people. Trying to prepare for those interactions stressed me out. I wanted to represent myself, my family, and Black women well. I couldn't wear sweatpants or look messy. I had to put on makeup, make sure my hair was covered or done and make sure my kids looked well taken care of. I had no idea how people there—whether patients or staff—would perceive me. It was a lot to think about on top of postpartum depression because I really didn't want to be there.

Navigating the healthcare system is not easy. When I first started seeking help, it would have been easier to simply say, "Forget this! Therapy's obviously not for me." At that time, I had never been to therapy. The first therapist stared at me with wide eyes as I shared my story. She seemed completely shocked, and I left feeling like I needed help that I couldn't receive.

Honestly, I felt like if I had been White, if I had experiences she could relate to, she may have been able to help me, but she couldn't. I had to search long and hard. I had to put in the search bar on the internet "Black therapists." I had a lot of ups and downs with my insurance company because I wanted a Black female therapist, but there were so few that it made it even more difficult to get help. I wanted someone who would listen, but I also wanted to see someone who looked like me. I started looking for ethnic names to find someone who might be able to identify with and help me.

Navigating the system also taught me that it's much easier for me to get help than it is for my brother, sons, or husband to find a therapist. They need a Black male therapist, and there are not many Black male therapists. On top of that, in the event they find one, there's no guarantee they will connect with him.

Her Healing

The first time around it was really hard to cope because I didn't understand what was happening to me. It wasn't until I went to therapy that I discovered I had depression—have always had it—and it worsened after giving birth. It was a lot to digest. It was a lot to understand and process. By the time I was pregnant for the second time, I had built a foundation, so coping was much easier for me. I knew my triggers, I understood when I was being triggered, and I had spiritual practices in place. I knew how and when to reach out to my support group and how to communicate my needs.

Having that foundation also helped me understand that my cup has to be full in order to see and help someone else. Before I learned this truth, my mindset was to take care of the baby and my husband, then take care of myself. My mindset has since shifted, and I now know I need to take care of myself so I can take care of my family. That's the key—understanding that I need to take care of myself first and that I have to give myself grace and be patient with myself.

As I think about my own healing, I am drawn to thinking about others who are dealing with depression. We all need to take care of ourselves, be patient with ourselves, and learn to deal with things, but that process is different for everyone.

I remember trying to cope in the beginning when I didn't know what to do or where to turn. The most difficult thing I had to do was choose to live. Each day, I struggled with the thought that everyone would be better off without me and that I was not contributing to this world. I don't recall the exact moment, but at some point, I became aware that all my emotions and physical ailments were cyclical, and the healing process never actually stops. We have to take accountability for ourselves and create the environment we need. No one else can do it for us. Therapy, a good spouse, amazing parents—none of that matters if we are not willing to do the work to take care of ourselves. Every day is an opportunity to heal, and the process never ends.

I had to learn to forgive myself for being an awful person to my husband. I had to stop questioning if he would want to be with someone like me, and I had to choose forgiveness and be vulnerable instead of building up walls. It was difficult, but once I realized who I was and how I could heal, I was able to better cope during my second pregnancy and after giving birth.

In spite of all the pain, all the difficulties coping and relearning who I am, in spite of being vulnerable and working through forgiveness, I MADE IT! That was my biggest triumph. All that we went through as a family brought us to the point where, in the midst of the Coronavirus pandemic, my husband and I are better than we've ever been. We lean on each other in a way that allows us to be more vulnerable with each other. We made it—*that's* my biggest victory. The feeling of victory let me know everything is going to be okay. I experience more good days than bad now, and I am not concerned if other people understand the tools I use to cope. I'm doing what I need to do in order to bring myself joy. When my son was born, I played Christmas music the first week just to get out of bed.

Sometimes I wish I could go back and speak with my younger self. I would let her know that everything she ever dreamed she wanted would come and be better than she ever imagined. I would tell my younger self, "Keep fighting for yourself. Don't stop advocating for yourself. Trust the universe. Trust God." Five years after giving birth to my first son, things are much better than I ever thought they would be.

I know there are many women going through the same thing I've experienced. I want to let you know that there is a light at the end of the tunnel if you choose to do the work, heal, and stay true to yourself. There is purpose in this life, and you are going to make a difference in your life, your child's life, and someone else's life. Your story is going to help someone else, but you cannot tell that story if you're not here. You can't share your life and help others do the work to heal if you're not here. Don't accept whatever is given to you. *Seek help and fight for the help you need instead of accepting what is given to you.*

I've learned a lot through my experiences with postpartum depression. I had two different experiences with two different pregnancies. I feel confident for my next pregnancy and the one after it. Postpartum depression is connected to giving birth, so I'm excited to see what happens after the baby making and baby birthing stages. I feel as though I am birthing more than children. I'm birthing so much that is connected to my health and healing, and I wonder what is going to happen in the next stages of my life.

Let's reflect upon Jamila's story. Postpartum depression can manifest differently among women (Centers for Disease Control and Prevention, 2020b). It is often characterized by feelings of anger, withdrawing from loved ones, crying more than usual, feeling numb or disconnected from the baby, feeling guilty about not being a good mom, or worrying that you will hurt the baby.

Postpartum depression has, for far too long, been swept under the rug. Often, Black women avoid talking about postpartum depression due to fear of embarrassment, stigma, and shame. We can no longer allow women to suffer in silence and feel alone in their struggle to overcome the mental challenges experienced after giving birth.

I applaud Jamila because even in her darkest moments of suicide ideation, she reached out for help. Professional mental health counseling is essential to your well-being. You know what else is important? Let's build a tribe around our pregnant sisters and new moms to support and comfort them. So often, they feel alone in their new journey. Be that warrior that they need!

A Warrior Named Symone:
Her Battle with Anxiety

Breathe, eat your Oreos, get back to loving you, and do what you need to do.
—Symone

Generalized anxiety disorder is one of the most common types of mental health disorders in the United States (Neal-Barnet, 2018; Anxiety and Depression Association of America, 2020). Women are twice as likely as men to experience generalized anxiety disorder (Watson, Roberts & Saunders, 2012). Although varying statistics regarding racial differences exist, when examining generalized anxiety disorder, Black women experience more intense symptoms than White women (Neal-Barnet, 2018; Anxiety and Depression Association of America, 2020). We spoke with Symone, a 31-year-old engaged Black woman, about anxiety. Let's learn from this warrior.

Her Definition

I define anxiety as not being able to relax or breathe, having racing thoughts, trying to figure out how to calm down, and stomach tightness.

Generalized anxiety disorders are emotions characterized by recurring thoughts and concerns, worry, and feelings of tension (National Institute of Mental Health, 2017; Barlow, 2020).

Her Experience

Being a mother to three Black children, a daughter to Black parents, a fiancée to a Black man, and a sister to Black brothers has influenced how I view the world when it comes to anxiety. With all of the things that are going on in the world, I get very anxious when I think about the Black men in my family. I worry about my fiancé and brothers due to police brutality against Black people, specifically Black men. I worry about whether my fiancé will make it back home when he leaves. If he were to get stopped by the police, would he be harassed, especially since he is tall, big, and outspoken? They could possibly end his life.

As a sister, I worry about my brothers being in similar situations. My youngest brother has an intellectual disability; therefore, I worry about him a lot since his disability is not visible. If my parents weren't here, and if I didn't take him in, where would he go? How would life affect him as a Black male with an intellectual disability?

I have similar concerns for my eldest son, who is 9 years old and also has an intellectual disability. I will never know what it is like to be a young Black boy who grows into a Black man with an intellectual disability that is not visible. I worry about my children constantly, and as the daughter of Black parents, I think about the socioeconomic status in the Black community and hope my parents can retire and live comfortably.

Although haunted by all of these thoughts, I didn't realize for a long time that I had anxiety coupled with postpartum depression. After I had my daughter in February 2018, I decided to call my healthcare provider. For months prior to calling my healthcare provider, I felt detached, and my emotions were up and down. I was in graduate school but felt like I couldn't do it. I would make up all types of excuses prior to studying or starting a project. If there was something around the house that needed to be done, I would make up all types of scenarios in my head. I didn't know where to start. I would just feel withdrawn and unorganized. When I went to my healthcare provider, they immediately put me on medication and referred me to counseling. They diagnosed me with anxiety and postpartum depression.

Thinking back, I believe my anxiety started when I had to return to work after maternity leave. I was working late nights at the post office and I was not ready to go back to work; however, I did not have a choice due to financial reasons. My fiancé and I were not permanent employees with benefits yet, so I had to go back and send my daughter to daycare. I thought I was ready, but I wasn't. I felt bad for not bonding as much as I wanted to with my daughter and my eldest son.

Her Well-Being

Recently, I've been having more conversations about how I'm affected by anxiety and postpartum depression. I often hear other women, including women in my family, talk about how they feel, and I ask them if they are okay and tell them to speak with a healthcare provider or therapist. In a way, it has influenced me to be more communicative and open. I realize that I am not alone when dealing with anxiety and other mental health issues.

Anxiety did take a toll on my mental and emotional health because I was also dealing with depression. At first, I used to feel like a messed-up person. I thought something was wrong with me. However, I will not let anxiety defeat me or define me. I'm not perfect. I am human. I am still a loving, kind person; God still loves me.

Therefore, I had to find myself. You know, I've always been the type to unwind by drinking tea and listening to music. I learned to journal and express myself by telling others that I am going through something. I would let people know that I have anxiety and depression and some days are just not good days for me.

Due to having anxiety and postpartum depression, I started snacking. I should also mention that I have PCOS. Therefore, my weight fluctuates. Being anxious about it doesn't help at all. Some days I will say, "You know what? I'm going to eat these Oreos, I'm going to own these Oreos, and I'm going to deal with the consequences tomorrow." Some days are not always going to be rainbows and unicorns and shit.

When I think about anxiety, I often think, "I can't do this." What I mean by that statement is that I can't schedule my week, my family's week, figure out how to go to work, and how to do school assignments. I feel so unorganized and overwhelmed. Moreover, my anxiety makes me worry about how I can spend time with family and friends.

Her Support System

Outside of my therapist, my main support system is my fiancé, mom, aunt, and dad. However, my fiancé is my main support system. Sometimes, I will tell my fiancé how I feel. He will call my mom or aunt, and they will come over.

In addition, I enjoy speaking with my therapist because she can help me see things. I also don't want to be a burden to my family; I want to take a load off of them and deal with my shit on my own.

However, there are aspects of my support system that could be improved. My first therapist was nice; however, I think she could have been a little more down-to-earth, like, "Okay, you need to get your shit together." She was communicative, but I just felt like okay, this is too glittery. After that experience, I looked for a Black therapist because I wanted someone with whom I could relate. Regardless of how or where Black women grew up, we can always relate to each other as Black women in general.

Her Intersection of Healthcare

In the healthcare system, I did not understand why the first thing they did was put me on medication. I always feel like that is what the healthcare system does. Moreover, at the time I had private insurance and state insurance. There were times when my Medicaid was not accepted. However, there were times when my therapist could not see me because my private insurance was not able to be billed. My private insurance did not cover mental health services. So imagine if I did not have my secondary insurance, I would not have been able to be treated. I wonder how many women don't have sufficient insurance to attend therapy. I also did teletherapy on days when I didn't want to get up and drive to sessions. I wonder if every woman has that luxury.

My most memorable moment in the healthcare system was a few months ago when I was at the OBGYN office with my nurse practitioner. When she came into the room, she had a student with her. She did my exam and asked me how I was doing. When they left the room, the door was still cracked. I overheard my nurse practitioner say, "This is a good day for her." She was talking about me! It made me take a look at myself. I wondered how I looked before, you know, before I started this journey of healing and seeing healthcare providers and my therapist. I wondered how they viewed me when I first met them. Did I look that crazy?

Her Healing

I've learned to cope by understanding that some days are not going to be good. That doesn't necessarily mean the entire day, maybe it's only a few moments, but I know that regardless I will be okay. I step back and breathe. That's what helped me. If I need a little more reinforcement, I will call my aunt or my fiancé or take a moment to think.

My biggest challenge when experiencing anxiety is that my head feels cloudy or I get a headache and need to nap in the middle of the day. My stress levels impact my anxiety. I'm a mom of three, with two little ones and a 9 year old. I want to spend more time with my children, so that's anxiety right there. I can't get rid of my babies, so what can I get rid of that's not bringing me peace and contributing to my anxiety? I had a job that I didn't care for, but I needed to work. You know, it wasn't even something that I went to school for. So what did I decide to do? I decided to get rid of that job.

My biggest triumph is telling myself it'll be okay. And feeling okay. I had to learn to relax. There was a turning point in my life regarding my anxiety that involved my son. My oldest son was used to me being withdrawn. I would often come home, go in my room, and close the door. One day, I had a headache and decided to lie down. I remember him standing at the top of the stairs looking at me as if he was scared of me. That was a turning point for me. I had to say, "Okay, you need to figure it out. Figure it out."

Thinking back, if I had to share pieces of advice with my younger self, I would share that it is okay to ask for help. Even if you think the problem is small, ask for help. Sometimes, we let our pride get in the way or think that we can figure it out on our own. You have to communicate, whether it's with a healthcare provider, friend, family member, or mentor.

My advice to other women who are in a similar situation is that it will be okay and they will be okay. You know, I'm still dealing with anxiety, but I'm not getting headaches, napping, or withdrawing from my children. I'm the happiest I have ever been. Seeking help and communicating more has really helped me. I had to learn how to communicate and how to ask for help. I also advise other women to *journal*, listen to music, drink tea, or whatever they need to do to feel better.

When I look at where I am now, I know it's getting better. I'm still dealing with it, but it's getting better.

Let's reflect upon Symone's story. Generalized anxiety disorder is emotions characterized by recurring thoughts and concerns, worry, and feelings of tension (National Institute of Mental Health, 2017; Barlow, 2020). Generalized anxiety disorder can manifest in individuals differently (Villines, 2020). Common symptoms include a racing heart; tension in the chest or butterflies in the stomach; feeling irritable or on edge; having trouble concentrating; and developing anxiety-related ailments, such as headaches or chronic muscle pain. What do you do when your head hurts, your mind races, your body sweats, and your heartbeat increases? What do you do when you feel like the weight of the world is upon your shoulders?

To understand Black women and generalized anxiety disorder, one must understand how the intersection of race, class, and gender influences mental health. The historical Black experience, composed of oppression and dehumanization caused by individual, institutional, and structural racism, has riddled the Black community with multiple layers of racial trauma that can contribute to anxiety (Mental Health America, 2021).

I applaud Symone for seeking professional mental health treatment. Due to fear, stigma, and mistrust of the healthcare system, Blacks are less likely to seek professional mental health services. One should note that when Black women do utilize mental health services, they want a therapist who understands them, their needs, and what it's like to be a Black woman in the United States. However, only about 4% of psychologists in the United States are Black (Floyd, 2020).

Nevertheless, do not allow that to discourage you from seeking help. Counseling will change your life and help you to become the best version of yourself. In life, some days will be more difficult than others, but allowing yourself grace and love will help you get through those tough times. Let's activate the warrior and fight like hell, understanding that you are not alone in this plight.

A WAR OF ABUSE AND VIOLENCE

A Warrior Named Sara:
Her Battle with Emotional Abuse

The best part about every morning you have a new opportunity to make a better and happier version of yourself.

—Sara

Black women experience several different types of abuse—for instance, emotional abuse—at significantly higher rates than their White counterparts (Green, 2017). Sara, a 30-year-old, married Black woman, experienced emotional abuse from her mother. Let's hear from this warrior and learn more about her experience.

Her Definition

Emotional abuse is defined as being distressed in a cage because others are trying to mold you into someone that you are not. It changes who you are emotionally, as if altering your genetic makeup, your DNA.

Emotional abuse is nonphysical behavior that is used to control, punish, or isolate an individual through fear, dominance, or humiliation (Karakurt & Silver, 2013). Often, emotional abuse precedes physical abuse.

Her Experience

Emotional abuse has decreased my confidence and self-esteem. It leaves holes inside you. I was damaged. I was sinking. It manifests into your reality. My emotional abuse started in childhood with my mother. Her way of showing love was tough love. There were things that I just couldn't tell her.

When my mother found out that I lost my virginity, she called me all types of names—as if I was a stranger—such as ho, slut, and bitch. It was not normal. Then she was like, "Well, if you get pregnant, it's on you to take care of it." I was not prepared for her reaction. I started second-guessing myself. Maybe I am a slut. Maybe I am that person. That event changed me a lot. That was my first experience with emotional abuse.

Her Well-Being

Emotional abuse has influenced my life as a Black woman because it's never enough, no matter what you do. You're also always second-guessing yourself. It's like you dive into an ocean, and it's so deep that there's no bottom to it. It's like an abyss. You're just sinking and sinking and sinking.

I believed that God was punishing me because I wasn't doing right. I lost my virginity, then I became interested in women. It was a domino effect. Would he forgive me? I had to eventually start viewing God differently and say, "God is love" and "God is patient."

I felt as if I didn't have good mental or emotional health. I felt like a robot. I felt as if I was missing a part of me. Like, "Okay Sara, you're missing a bolt." The bolt is self-confidence. What's happening on the inside reflects on the outside. I was experiencing bags under my eyes and bouts of depression. You could see it all over my face. You could see it in my eyes, and of course, you know the old saying, your eyes are the windows to your soul.

When I think about emotional abuse, three experiences come to mind. The first one is when my mother found out that I lost my virginity. The second experience was with my first boyfriend. He cheated on me so many times. He cheated on me and told me to my face that he cheated on me. It was like he was telling me that I'm not good enough because I wouldn't do what he wanted me to do. The third experience was not setting boundaries in college. By not setting boundaries, I was emotionally abused by people who I thought were my friends.

The feelings that I have when I experience emotional abuse compare to lying on railroad tracks. I'm lying there but not tied down. I'm just lying there. The train is coming, and I'm not moving. I know it's there. I know it's coming my direction, but I'm still lying there. My emotions are telling me that I'm trapped. I'm tied down. Not physically, but I'm tied down. I'm hesitant to move. I know it's coming. I see it, but my body will not move. That's how powerful the mind is.

Her Support System

My current support system is my wife, her sister, and my new friends. I really want to add a therapist because of the scars. I, as a Black woman, have so many scars. My supporters are honest with me. They let me know that I am human, that it's okay to feel the way that I feel, that it's okay to break down. They also let me know that I don't have to just accept breaking down; it can be fixed. They encouraged me to start over, to be grounded, to stand on a solid foundation. However, I am very timid; therefore, communication can always be improved. You know, I may be uncomfortable but that does not mean someone's efforts are not reaching me.

Her Healing

I am learning how to cope with my emotional abuse. It's a learning process. I had to look within myself and say, "No matter what changes around me, as long as I am who I am and have a solid foundation, that's all that matters." My biggest challenge with emotional abuse was my pride. I was like, "Fuck that—I'm okay, I'm strong." No, I'm not strong. Or, "I'm okay, I'm good," but I wasn't good. However, my biggest triumph was my haircut. I was so attached to my hair because it's who I am. I shaved my hair off. It was so much mayhem and wildfires in my life that I just needed to clear everything and start over.

My turning point was when my wife was telling me that she was tired. She was like, "Baby, I have held you down since we've been together, I'm tired." And I was like, "Girl, you tired?" I had to step up. I had to stand on my own two feet.

If I had to have a conversation with my younger self, I would tell my younger self that people will come and go like seasons. I would tell my younger self to see a therapist and talk about emotions. I have improved by leaps and bounds, but there's still more work to be done.

Now, let's reflect. Emotional abuse, which may include verbal assault, control, ridicule, or use of intimate knowledge for degradation, influences the emotional, mental, and psychological well-being of an individual (Karakurt & Silver, 2013). It can often leave individuals feeling confused, hopeless, and ashamed.

One thing about abuse, specifically emotional abuse, is that we must address it head on in order to prevent it from manifesting in other relationships and areas of our lives. When you experience emotional abuse, you are more likely to allow others to continuously abuse you. It's a traumatic cycle that must be broken.

I am encouraged by Sara's story. She provided information that most of us wouldn't have felt comfortable sharing. As we close the discussion, it is important to understand Sara's experiences. Sara experienced childhood emotional abuse from her mother and emotional abuse in relationships and friendships. Sara is finding her strength through healing.

Have you been in situations that have left you scarred? That have left you feeling as if you are not enough? Well, I am here to tell you, you are enough. You are more than enough.

You are enough in all that you do.

So often, we try to hold on to people who are no longer meant to serve us. Evaluate situations that don't serve you and make you feel less than about yourself. Sometimes it's hard to walk away, but it's even harder finding yourself after you've lost yourself. Protect yourself by having boundaries. Boundaries are meant to protect you and your emotional, mental, spiritual, and physical well-being. We need to stop allowing everyone access to us, especially when they do not deserve it.

A Warrior Named Anjani:
Her Battle with Intimate Partner Violence

Leave, because your life depends on it.
—Anjani

Intimate partner violence against Black women is a major public health concern. Research has revealed that 45.1% of Black women have experienced intimate partner violence, and 51.3% of Black female homicides are due to intimate partner violence (National Coalition Against Domestic Violence, 2020). When compared to White women, Black women are three times more likely to die from intimate partner violence, making it one of the leading causes of death for Black women (Centers for Disease Control and Prevention, 2019). Anjani, a 36-year-old Black woman experienced intimate partner violence. This warrior's experiences provide us a better understanding of intimate partner violence.

Her Definition

Intimate partner violence is violence that occurs inside the home. Intimate partner violence comes in many forms, such as physical, verbal, mental or emotional abuse.

As defined by the Centers for Disease Control and Prevention (2021), intimate partner violence, which is characterized by physical violence, sexual violence, stalking, or psychological harm, occurs between current or former partners or spouses.

Her Experience

My childhood influenced how I navigate the world in regard to intimate partner violence. I grew up in a hostile environment, and the abuse began at a young age, which has influenced my choices as an adult. I chose men who behaved the same way and did the same things to me that were done to me during my childhood. It was psychological; the behavior became part of my subconscious, and I not only became used to it, I thought it was love. I had very low self-esteem, and after giving birth to my second child, I believed I didn't deserve anyone worthwhile. At that point, I felt like I had already become a statistic: multiple kids by multiple men and not married. According to society, I was only going to be good for sex. It was embedded in me.

I've been in four serious relationships, and I've had a child out of each one of those relationships, and three of those relationships were physically violent. The fourth relationship was only violent once. He did not strike me like the other men, but the relationship was still hostile.

My first experience with intimate partner violence was with my eldest child's father. This was my shortest relationship as an adult. He and I met in college, and when I got pregnant, I dropped out of school. He would stay out all night, only coming into the house around 5 a.m. At that point in our relationship, I started talking to other guys because I felt like he was cheating on me. He always came home in the wee hours of the morning, so it seemed evident to me that he was unfaithful.

When my son was 5 months old, things became violent. I was going to my friend's wedding and did not want him to go. However, he was still getting dressed to go. He went into the bedroom, looked through my phone, and saw I was talking to other guys when he was out all night. He turned and threw my son's bottle at me. The bottle hit my son and me and burst. When I got up, he slammed me onto a chair and choked me until I passed out. When I came to, I was able to get to my phone and text a friend to come over. While she was there, he choked me again and threw me on the bed. While pinned down on the bed, I headbutted him and was able to get free and climb out of the window.

Believe it or not, I still went to the wedding because I had nowhere else to go. While I was sitting down at the wedding, someone tapped me on the shoulder. I turned around, and it was him. My face flushed with pure terror. After the wedding, several of my girlfriends asked what happened, and after I finished explaining, they were adamant that I leave right away. He still showed up to the reception, but they were all ready to fight him. He kept saying he needed me, that he needed my son and me, but that day was the end of our relationship.

My next abusive relationship was with my eldest daughter's father. He was crazy—by far the craziest one. When he "found" God, he became violent. One day, he tried to prevent me from coming into the house. After I got into the house, we started fighting like two men in the street. He pushed me to the ground, smashed a Bible in my face, and told me I was the devil. I was pregnant at the time, so I started vomiting uncontrollably. Our daughter, who was 1 year old at the time, was crying. I went into the bedroom to get her; he grabbed my ankle and snatched me off the bed while I was holding her. But here's the kicker, the next day he proposed.

The violent relationship continued, but I had nowhere to go. I had alienated myself from my friends and family. When I finally got the courage to leave, he and his mother tried to fight me in the kitchen. Both my kids were hanging onto my legs. I ended up homeless with two kids and decided to have an abortion.

It got crazier from there. After I had finally moved into a new apartment, I opened the door to leave one day, and he punched me in the face, grabbed my daughter, and took off. I tried to get my daughter out of the car, but he started fighting me like I was a man. I was no match for his strength.

My third abusive relationship was with my second daughter's father. He was the most insecure and jealous of them all. The abuse started when I went out with my best friend for her birthday. I posted pictures on social media and he got upset. He said that I was smiling more in the pictures with her than I did with him. He punched me and we started fighting. The next day he proposed, just like the other men I'd been with. Because of my low self-esteem, I agreed and said yes. By this time, I had three kids by three different men and didn't think I could get anyone else at that point.

While I said yes to the proposal, the abuse continued. I woke up to him standing over me. Everything in that relationship was a fight. He was extremely disrespectful and not only physically abusive but verbally abusive to me in front of my kids. Eventually, I left and called off the wedding. He was not afraid to beat on me, so I knew I had to go. I had miscarried a child due to the abuse.

My last abusive relationship was with my youngest daughter's father. I thought he was different, but he revealed that he was the same as the other men. He never struck me as they did, but when the relationship ended, he called me hateful things in front of my children. He called me a dummy, which I hate because I was called that when I was younger. He called me bitch and ho, just really provoking the situation. He closed the door in my face and it nicked my nose, so we started fighting. We had people over, and they made him leave, and that is how the relationship ended. He hasn't changed, though. We've been broken up for 3 years. I saw him 2 days ago, and he told me that he was going to beat my ass and beat the ass of the man I was dating.

Her Well-Being

When it comes to relationships, I have trust issues. I am scared that someone will present himself to be a nice, stand-up guy but then try to control me. I don't let anyone get close to me, and it is hard for me to trust a man who says he wants to love me but not control me. I am always waiting for the other shoe to drop. To be honest, this is the first time in my adult life that I have been single. I have been in a relationship since I was 16 years old. I'm sure the way I was raised has had a great influence on my outlook. I was abandoned by both parents, beat on by my family, and my brother was killed.

One thing many people don't know about me is that, since college, I have taken comfort in the practices of Buddhism because Buddhists don't believe in God or gods. Buddhism focuses on you, your energy, and how that energy comes back to you. I've been surrounded by Christians all my life, and the ones who have hurt me the most have been Christians. Due to the hurt, I steer clear of Christianity. Now, everything I do is based on energy, walking the righteous path, and living a righteous life. As long as I am doing right by myself and my children, then right will come to me. I don't give God the credit, though. Anything I do, I feel like I do because of me, and I deserve the credit. I don't even mention my beliefs to others because once I say what I believe, they look at me like I'm crazy. Most people don't know anything about Buddhism, so they assume I worship serpents with six heads and weird gods. I don't like talking about spirituality because people are not as open-minded as they say.

Intimate partner violence has influenced my mental and emotional health as a Black woman because on the outside looking in, I'm the strongest person you'll ever meet. However, to be honest, I am very fragile and broken. I won't show emotion because I fear it will be used against me. Even my kids see me as a robot—you know, nothing hurts me and nothing makes me angry. The truth is everything makes me angry. I don't allow anyone to see my raw emotions unless I'm provoked in the moment. Instead of getting upset, I simply walk away.

Due to the stress, I developed ulcerative colitis. Physically, the violence took a toll on my body. When most people think of physical violence, they think of black eyes, bruises, and maybe broken bones, but it's more than that. Now, I deal with depression from time to time. I can't even date freely because my exes are always nearby. I turn around, and there they are. They show up unexpectedly and pop up at my house asking to see their kids. I can't get the space I require. They have no boundaries, no matter how hard I try to create them. It is overwhelming, but because I hide my emotions, people do not know what I'm going through.

It is a very strange experience getting beat up and then proposed to the next day. Men are impulsive when they are angry. The first thing they do once the dust settles is apologize or make a grand gesture. The gestures were consistent—gifts, engagement proposals, cars, and flowers sent to my school or job. And yes, one of them literally beat me and proposed the next day with a ring that looked like it came from a bubblegum machine. With all of the guys, I took a lot of abuse before it became physical—tons of verbal, mental, and emotional abuse. When it became physical, that was always the breaking point for me. I just had to figure out how to leave without causing more drama. I always saw things on TV that scared me and made me think he was going to kill me. Every time I've been physically abused by a man I thought that in that moment he was going to kill me.

I remember being alone. Scared and helpless with nowhere to go. Sometimes I wanted to die. Those are the feelings I had. If I didn't have children, there would have been no reason for me to live. I'm no stranger to trying to commit suicide. There is no doubt that the only reason I'm alive today is because of my children.

Her Support System

I did not have a support system. When I had the opportunity to move out and get my own place, I distanced myself from my entire family. As a child, my family caused much harm to me. Some of them even turned a blind eye to my abuse. It had been 2 years since I moved out before they started to find out what happened to me as a child. Since I didn't have anyone around, when I left one abuser, the only place I had to go was to another abuser. I really had nowhere to go.

If I had a support system, things might have been different. I may have been more vocal. However, I realized that people watched the shit get beat out of me as a child and never stepped in. If they didn't help then, why would they help now? It took me years to reach out for help because I thought that people would blame me for being in those situations and label me a statistic.

Her Healing

I coped by covering everything up, even as a child. Growing up, I was embarrassed; my best friends didn't even know what was going on. I was too embarrassed to speak up, which caused me to hold in everything. It caused me to shut down and made it difficult to ask for help.

Things would have been different for me if I had seen the signs prior to getting into a relationship with them. However, my self-esteem was so low and I was filled with so many insecurities that I went for the first guy who showed me attention. What's crazy is that all four of the men who abused me watched their own mother get beat, and most of their fathers were on drugs. I didn't ask the right questions. I didn't notice the red flags.

My biggest triumph is still being here, I am a winner. I am not where I want to be, but I am not where I used to be. I push through because of my children. Someone once told me that once I get to the place in life I want to be, I'm not going to credit myself, I'm going to give all the credit to my children. They are right.

With my second daughter's father, I started to gain strength to say enough is enough. I was subjected to every form of abuse that you could imagine. Now, I was never the one to sit there and take a beating, I most definitely fought back, but I was tired of fighting. I was tired of being beat. When I lost the baby, that was a huge turning point for me. I kept telling myself that my children could not see the abuse. In addition, he was starting to be mean to my older children. I knew I had to move on.

If I could share any advice with my younger self, it would be to get to know the men you date. Moreover, if you are struggling with insecurities and low self-esteem, work on you first before getting into a relationship. Love yourself, know your worth, appreciate the person you are. I had to realize that while I do have four children by four different men, that does not make me less of a woman.

I want to encourage all women in intimate partner relationships to leave as soon as you can. Do not wait until it gets worse. Ladies, the first time you get an inkling that he doesn't respect you, LEAVE. Women give people the benefit of the doubt too much, even when people show us exactly who they are. We cannot change people, and we do not owe anyone an explanation for doing what is best for us. Don't walk around scared of what *might happen*. If you believe it *could happen*, leave quietly.

As I reflect upon where I am now, I am happy to share my story. I believe my experiences caused me to be stronger, but my experiences have also let people see that if I can make it, they can make it as well. Someone needs to hear about how someone else made it through. I never heard anyone else's story. I was alone, making it however I could, but if I could have found the courage to express what I was going through sooner, I may have found support in other places. My story is no longer mine to hold on to and keep private; it is mine to share and help others.

Let's reflect upon Anjani's story. Black women are disproportionately affected by intimate partner violence (Green, 2017). One must question, how do the interactions of gender and race contribute to high rates of intimate partner violence? The answer is Black women occupy multiple marginalized identities. The violence against Black women has occurred for far too long. This violence is rooted in the history of slavery and oppression, which can be traced to how slave masters treated Black women.

Research has noted that Black women may create a "strong" façade as a mental and emotional health protective factor (West et al., 2016) However, this may have a crippling effect on Black women's mental and emotional health. Have you ever used the strong facade? Have you ever felt fragile? Have you ever felt broken?

Setting personal boundaries is important to not only your spiritual, mental, and physical health, but as in Anjani's situation, your physical health as well. Personal boundaries set the tone, basic guidelines, and stipulations for what you require, how you expect others to treat you, and who you allow in your space. Anjani's number one rule for personal boundaries is, "If it costs me my peace, let it go."

I commend Anjani for this advice. So often we as women, specifically Black women, stay in expired situations that don't serve us. We stay because of love and loyalty, but ladies, we must learn to love ourselves first. And the first step of that is leaving. I am encouraged by Anjani sharing her most vulnerable and authentic self with us. I am empowered by her bravery and strength. She is a warrior, a warrior who fought to find her healing!

A Warrior Named Brenda:
Her Battle with Sexual Abuse

Pain only lasts so long before it manifests into magnificence.
—Brenda

The fight to protect Black women has been a struggle since slavery (Barlow, 2020), specifically due to the objectification and exploitation of the Black body (Cooper, 2015). Black women slaves were dehumanized, raped, sexually coerced, and forced to reproduce children fathered by their slave owner (National Organization for Women, 2018). Now, fast forward to 2021, and Black women still remain vulnerable to sexual violence (Barlow, 2020). Thirty-five percent of Black women experience some form of sexual violence in their lifetime (Barlow, 2020), so now let's hear from a warrior named Brenda, a 40-year-old Black woman, to learn more about her experience with sexual violence.

Her Definition

Sexual violence is defined as any physical contact without consent.

Sexual violence is any sexual activity without obtained or freely given consent (Centers for Disease Control and Prevention, 2021).

Her Experience

When someone experiences sexual violence at a young age, it manifests into adulthood. Therefore, as a mother, I pay attention to my daughters' changes in behavior. I ensure that I ask questions and have conversations about sexual violence. I'm probably a little strict.

My earliest memories of sexual violence were when I was 5 years old and molested by a teenage family member. He was inappropriately touching me; however, no penetration occurred. As a child, we used to visit this family member's house. The adults would send the kids off to play. I was excited to play because I came from poverty, and he had the most incredible room. While playing with his toys, he asked me if I wanted to sit on his lap. I remember thinking—at 5 years old—*Someone wants to treat me like a baby again.* I went to sit on his lap, and I remember his hand going up my shirt; it was uncomfortable.

My second experience with sexual violence happened at a sleepover when I was 11 years old. A close family friend raped me. This event was very traumatic.

My experiences with sexual violence are why I have been in therapy. I often told myself that I allowed it. Therapy made me realize that I was 5 years old and could not have prevented it. Due to the sexual violence, I grew up enamored with him because I interpreted his actions as an expression of love. Like, oh, somebody wants to be around me. From that day forward, I followed him around incessantly and sought his attention.

Her Well-Being

Sexual violence taught me that I did not have a voice or that my voice did not matter. I didn't realize how much it impacted me as a Black woman. However, I knew how it affected me as a woman, and of course, as a little girl, but as a Black woman, we are judged in ways that I do not see with our White counterparts or races and ethnicities. Often, people act like sexual violence is rare; however, it is prevalent in our community.

Ultimately, the abuse I suffered caused me to walk away from spirituality completely. I didn't believe that a higher being or higher power would allow something like that to happen. I recently just regained my spirituality again about 5 years ago.

Sexual violence has intensified my struggle as a Black woman. It creates more distrust, anger, and sadness. Everything that I was destined to feel as a Black woman was intensified by being vulnerable due to my past. As a result, I gained weight out of fear of attracting people. I didn't want to be attractive. I didn't want to be desired. I thought that no one would want me if I packed on the pounds.

I often think about past experiences. The experience that comes to mind was my first encounter with sexual violence when I was 5 years old. I often wonder, what could I have done differently? Did I say something? Did I do something? The second experience that comes to mind is rape. I go back to that day regularly because it exemplified a behavior pattern. There was a part of me that was broken. Over the years, I have spent a lot of time consoling myself and reliving the experience to try and move beyond it. The third experience that comes to mind is the first time I willingly had sex at 26 years old. To clarify, I'm not saying that everyone I had sex with prior to that experience was rape, but I am saying that I had the mindset that I was not allowed to say no. When someone wanted to have sex, I said yes and had sex. When I think back, I remember the difference in the encounter and realize the difference between what I experienced before and what I experienced then. I was able to make a conscious decision about what I wanted to do. Sexual abuse is like drowning. You can't breathe. Even thinking about it now, I can't breathe.

Her Support System

My support system was nonexistent. I was raped at 11 years old while at a close family member's sleepover. My uncle watched it happen through the window. He told my mom, "Hey, I saw Brenda having sex." My mom never asked me about the situation. Instead, she immediately stated that I would be just like my grandmother and told me if I needed to get on birth control to let her know. If she had only asked me, I would've told her. She didn't even ask me.

If I found out that my 11-year-old daughter was having sex, I would have had a conversation with her, you know, asking questions, such as, "What were you doing? Where did you learn that?" There was never a conversation. It wasn't until I was 18 years old that I told my mom about what happened. So, yeah, there was no support system.

I went through years of emotional damage and mental anguish. All they had to do was ask me. All they had to do was ask me a question. Now, my mom is very defensive about it. However, I was 11 years old. I implore people to ask. That's why I never told anyone. No one asked. I learned the importance of asking the people who I care about in my life precise questions.

Her Healing

I am still coping. I am usually fine; however, I have learned to identify my triggers. I am learning that there are broken pieces in me, and those broken pieces may sound good and look good, even though I know better. Therefore, I need to ensure that I can identify the things that speak to the broken parts of me for my mental and emotional health. I believe that's what helps me cope, you know, taking time to identify my triggers. I also journal. I am learning ways to navigate my experiences with sexual violence so it doesn't necessarily come out when I'm triggered.

My biggest challenge is forgiving those who sexually abused me. I often wonder if I can forgive them. If given the opportunity to do something to them, would I? I had to realize that's not necessarily true forgiveness. We hear so much that forgiveness is for you, and that's true. It's not for the other person. However, I understand that not forgiving is also allowed as long as I don't beat myself up about it. It can be healthy to keep me out of that situation.

My biggest triumph was overcoming, being resilient, and using the one thing meant to defeat me as a platform to catapult me. I can have conversations with clients and say, look at me, I'm not perfect. I have plenty of things that I work on daily, but being a beacon of light and letting someone know that they can overcome and get beyond sexual violence has been one of my triumphs.

I have experienced a lot of trauma, especially at a very young age. My adverse childhood experience (ACE) score is 10. By the time I was 7 years old, my ACE score was 7. There was a point in my life when my mental health was severely impacted. I would have panic attacks. At that time, I had three children, and they needed me. When I realized that, that was a turning point for me. I had to tell myself, "Yes, you experienced this. Yes, it sucked. Yes, it was awful. But, you have three other people you have to live for." I think I was like 19 years old when that happened.

I have written letters to my younger self. When I think back to the trauma that I have experienced, I always think I should have known what not to do or say, so I share that life is full of experiences that are meant to teach us something. It's always hard at the moment to figure out what they may be. However, we must take whatever preventive measures necessary to ensure our safety.

If you are waiting for the pain to go away, you'll be waiting forever. The pain does not go away. It changes. It shifts. It moves into different parts of our psyche, but it does not go away.

I float between absolute freedom and making sure I'm not doing things that speak to the broken parts of me. I have freedom now about sex that I've never experienced before. I also realize that abstaining is a type of freedom too. So, I can be open and free, or I can be closed and free. It goes either way; it is my choice.

There is so much secrecy in the Black community. I believe secrecy is embedded to prevent judgment from others. I don't need another thing for somebody to judge me on. That judgment feeds the secrecy, which creates a lack of support, empathy, and the ability to move forward.

Let's examine Brenda's story. One in four Black girls will experience sexual violence before the age of 18 years old (Barlow, 2020). Ninety percent of the time, children who experience sexual violence know the perpetrator of the abuse (National Sexual Violence Resource Center, 2010). The majority of Black women often are sexually assaulted at a young age and typically by a family member (Barlow, 2020). Moreover, prior unaddressed sexual violence leaves Black girls vulnerable to additional abuse and violence.

Sexual violence against Black women is a pervasive issue that is often unreported and underaddressed due to the stigma that is associated with it (National Sexual Violence Resource Center, 2010). Although some people may act as if sexual violence in Black women is rare, 35% of Black women experience some form of sexual violence (Barlow, 2020). Unfortunately, that's only the percentage of Black women who report their experience. Thirty-five percent! Imagine standing in a room of 100 Black women; approximately 35 of them have experienced sexual violence.

There are many reasons people who experience sexual violence do not report it. Some of the reasons include not being asked, shame and embarrassment, fear of not being believed, concern of being blamed, pressure to not tell, and desire to protect the perpetrator (National Sexual Violence Resource Center, 2010).

In Brenda's interview, she mentioned ACEs, which are traumatic events such as sexual violence that occur in childhood (0–17 years) and have an impact on chronic illness, mental health, future violence victimization and perpetration, and opportunity (Centers for Disease

Control and Prevention, 2020d). Sixty-one percent of Blacks have experienced at least one ACE (Sacks & Murphey, 2018).

I appreciate Brenda's vulnerability in sharing her story. I pray that this chapter helps the invisible suffering that many Black women endure. I am encouraged by Brenda's vulnerability. I applaud Brenda for seeking counseling to find peace and healing.

THE END OF A WAR

Conclusion

Throughout these chapters, we noticed differences in health outcomes that are not solely due to genetics, cultural factors, or behaviors; rather, these race-related health disparities are a physical manifestation of racism and discrimination in this country (Donnelly et al. 2020). These differences in health outcomes are rooted in the historical Black experience of individual, institutional, and structural racism (Mental Health America, 2021). The fight to protect Black women physically, mentally, emotionally, and spiritually has been a struggle, and for this reason, many Black women continue to suffer in silence due to the fact that Black women occupy the intersection of multiple marginalized identities, and these intersecting identities are woven through interconnected experiences.

These interconnected experiences are not individual but rather communal, especially in regard to the lack of effective patient-provider communication in Black women. Effective patient-provider communication is essential to promote improved health outcomes. Since Black women are more likely to experience inadequate patient-provider communication, we must advocate for ourselves by asking questions, seeking clarification, asking for a second opinion, knowing our rights, and doing our own research.

In addition, you can advocate for yourself by conversing with other women, specifically Black women, about their experiences. As demonstrated throughout these chapters, so often we experience similar circumstances yet do not have conversations with others out of fear, shame, and stigma.

However, there isn't anything to be ashamed about because throughout life we will experience difficult circumstances. We must understand that those difficult circumstances allow us to shed the broken and dead parts of us and to reemerge as the rising phoenix. Although you may feel abandoned, defeated, and frustrated, know that you are a season away from your rebirth.

You are the author and illustrator of your story. You have the power to write the introduction, middle, and ending of every chapter in your life. You control your final narrative. Everything that was sent and meant to destroy you has no power unless you allow it to define you.

Telling your story allows you to remove strongholds; break the generational curse of fear, shame, and stigma; and help other women who are in similar situations. Telling your story gives you the power to use your voice and to rise up against traumas you've suffered or obstacles in your life. Using your voice is what defines you as a warrior!

Remember, you are powerful, you are amazing, you are worthy, you are loved, you are valued, and your light shines brightly. Your story will serve as a testimony to other women. It takes courage and strength to walk in your truth and be true to yourself.

You are the embodiment of strength, tenacity, and perseverance. You are filled with purpose, walk in authority, and overflow with abundance. You are a warrior! A warrior who fought to find her healing!

.

REFERENCES

Alexander, L. L., LaRosa, J. H., Bader, H., Garfield, S., & Alexander, W. J. (2017). *New dimensions in women's health* (7th ed.). Jones and Bartlett Learning.

Anxiety and Depression Association of America. (2020). *Black community.* https://adaa.org/find-help/by-demographics/black-community

Barlow, J. N. (2020, February). Black women, the forgotten survivors of sexual assault. *In the Public Interest.* https://www.apa.org/pi/about/newsletter/2020/02/black-women-sexual-assault

Breast Cancer Prevention Partners. (2021). *At a glance.* https://www.bcpp.org/resource/african-american-women-and-breast-cancer/

Carbado, D. W., Crenshaw, K. W., Mays, V. M., & Tomlinson, B. (2013). Intersectionality: Mapping the movements of a theory. *Du Bois Review: Social Science Research on Race, 10*(2), 303–312. https://doi.org/10.1017/S1742058X13000349

Centers for Disease Control and Prevention. (2019). *Leading causes of death-females-non-Hispanic Black-United States, 2016.* https://www.cdc.gov/women/lcod/2016/nonhispanic-black/index.htm

Centers for Disease Control and Prevention. (2020a). *Breast cancer statistics.* https://www.cdc.gov/cancer/breast/statistics/

Centers for Disease Control and Prevention. (2020b). *Depression among women.* https://www.cdc.gov/reproductivehealth/depression/index.htm

Centers for Disease Control and Prevention. (2020c). *Infant mortality.* https://www.cdc.gov/reproductivehealth/maternalinfanthealth/infantmortality.htm

Centers for Disease Control and Prevention (2020d). *Preventing adverse childhood experiences.* https://www.cdc.gov/violenceprevention/aces/fastfact.html?CDC_AA _refVal=https%3A%2F%2Fwww.cdc.gov%2Fviolenceprevention%2Fa cestudy%2Ffastfact.html

Centers for Disease Control and Prevention. (2021). *Sexual violence.* https://www.cdc.gov/violenceprevention/sexualviolence/index.html

Cerezo, A., Cummings, M., Holmes, M., & Williams, C. (2020). Identity as resistance: Identity formation at the intersection of race, gender identity, and sexual orientation. *Psychology of Women Quarterly, 44*(1), 67-83. https://doi.org/10.1177/0361684319875977

Cleveland Clinic. (2020, February 20). *Can PCOS cause weight gain?* https://health.clevelandclinic.org/can-polycystic-ovary-syndrome-make-gain-weight/

Cooper, I. (2015). Commodification of the Black body, sexual objectification and social hierarchies during slavery. *Earlham Historical Journal, 7*(2), 21-43.

Donnelly, E., Dau, K. Q., Wilson-Mitchell, K., & Wren, J. I. (2020). Racism and health disparities. In K. D. Schuilng & L. E. Frances (Eds.), *Gynecologic health care: With an introduction to prenatal and postpartum care* (pp. 13-37). Jones & Bartlett Learning.

Echols, A. (2019, August 15). The challenges of breastfeeding as a Black person. *ACLU.* https://www.aclu.org/blog/womens-rights/pregnancy-and-parenting-discrimination/challenges-breastfeeding-black-person

Ely, D. M., & Driscoll, A. K. (2019). Infant mortality statistics, 2017: Data from the period linked birth/infant death file. *National Vital Statistics Reports, 68*(10), 1-19 https://www.cdc.gov/nchs/data/nvsr/nvsr68/nvsr68_10-508.pdf

Ely, D. M., & Driscoll, A. K. (2020). Infant mortality in the United States, 2018: Data from the period linked birth/infant death file. *National Vital Statistics Reports, 69*(7), 1-17.

Evans, N., Hsu, Y. L., & Sheu, J. J. (2021). Path model validation of breastfeeding intention among pregnant women. *JOGNN: Journal of Obstetric Gynecologic and Neonatal Nursing, 50*(2), 167-180. https://doi.org/10.1016/j.jogn.2020.10.007

Green, S. (2017, July 13). Violence against Black women: Many types, far-reaching effects. *Institute for Women's Policy Research.* https://iwpr.org/iwpr-issues/race-ethnicity-gender-and-economy/violence-against-black-women-many-types-far-reaching-effects/

Grey, H. (2020, November 23). *Black women, fibroids, and heavy bleeding.* Healthline. https://www.healthline.com/health/womens-health/black-women-and-heavy-periods

Howell, E. A., Mora, P. A., Horowitz, C. R., & Leventhal, H. (2005). Racial and ethnic differences in factors associated with early postpartum depressive symptoms. *Obstetrics and Gynecology, 105*(6), 1442–1450. https://doi.org/10.1097/01.AOG.0000164050.34126.37

Karakurt, G., & Silver, K. E. (2013). Emotional abuse in intimate relationships: The role of gender and age. *Violence and Victims, 28*(5), 804-821. https://doi.org/10.1891/0886-6708.vv-d-12-00041

Li, R., Perrine, C. G., Anstey, E. H., Chen, J., MacGowan, C. A., & Elam-Evans, L. D. (2019). Breastfeeding trends by race/ethnicity among US children born from 2009 to 2015. *JAMA Pediatrics, 173*(12), e193319. https://doi.org/10.1001/jamapediatrics.2019.3319

Mayo Clinic. (2020, October 03). *Polycystic ovary syndrome (PCOS)*. https://www.mayoclinic.org/diseases-conditions/pcos/symptoms-causes/syc-20353439

McKinney, C. O., Hahn-Holbrook, J., Chase-Lansdale, P. L., Ramey, S. L., Krohn, J., Reed-Vance, M., Raju, T. N., Shalowitz, M. U., & Community Child Health Research Network (2016). Racial and ethnic differences in breastfeeding. *Pediatrics, 138*(2), e20152388. https://doi.org/10.1542/peds.2015-2388

MedlinePlus. (2020). *Polycystic ovary syndrome*. https://medlineplus.gov/polycysticovarysyndrome.html

Morgan, T. (2016, March 20). Polycystic ovary syndrome (PCOS): What you don't know, but should. *BlackDoctor.Org*. https://blackdoctor.org/what-is-pcos/

Mostafavi, B. (2020, August 12). *Understanding racial disparities for women with uterine fibroids*. Michigan Medicine Health Lab. https://labblog.uofmhealth.org/rounds/understanding-racial-disparities-for-women-uterine-fibroids

Mukherjee, S., Velez Edwards, D. R., Baird, D. D., Savitz, D. A., & Hartmann, K. E. (2013). Risk of miscarriage among black women and white women in a US prospective cohort study. *American Journal of Epidemiology, 177*(11), 1271-1278. https://doi.org/10.1093/aje/kws393

National Coalition Against Domestic Violence. (2020). *Domestic violence and the Black community*. https://assets.speakcdn.com/assets/2497/dv_in_the_black_community.pdf

National Institute of Child Health and Human Development. (2017). *About pregnancy*. https://www.nichd.nih.gov/health/topics/pregnancy/conditioninfo

National Organization for Women Foundation. (2018). *Black women and sexual violence*. https://now.org/wp-content/uploads/2018/02/Black-Women-and-Sexual-Violence-6.pdf

National Partnership for Women and Families. (2018). *Black women's maternal health: A multifaceted approach to addressing persistent and dire health disparities*. https://www.nationalpartnership.org/our-work/health/reports/black-womens-maternal-health.html

National Sexual Violence Resources Center. (2010). *What is sexual violence?* https://www.nsvrc.org/sites/default/files/Publications_NSVRC_Factsheet_What-is-sexual-violence_1.pdf

Neal-Barnett, A. (2018, April 23). To be female, anxious and Black. *ADAA*. https://adaa.org/learn-from-us/from-the-experts/blog-posts/consumer/be-female-anxious-and-black

Office on Women's Health. (2019a). *Polycystic ovary syndrome*. https://www.womenshealth.gov/a-z-topics/polycystic-ovary-syndrome

Office on Women's Health. (2019b). *Postpartum depression*. https://www.womenshealth.gov/mental-health/mental-health-conditions/postpartum-depression

Sacks, V., & Murphey, D. (2018). *The prevalence of adverse childhood experiences, nationally, by state, and by race or ethnicity*. Child Trends. https://www.childtrends.org/publications/prevalence-adverse-childhood-experiences-nationally-state-race-ethnicity

Sandoiu, A. (2020, July 17). Postpartum depression in women of color: More work needs to be done. *Medical News Today*. https://www.medicalnewstoday.com/articles/postpartum-depression-in-women-of-color-more-work-needs-to-be-done#1

Spates, K., Evans, N. T., James, T. A., & Martinez, K. (2020). Gendered Racism in the lives of Black women: A qualitative exploration. *Journal of Black Psychology, 46*(8), 583-606. https://doi.org/10.1177/0095798420962257

Spates, K., Na'Tasha, M. E., Watts, B. C., Abubakar, N., & James, T. (2019). Keeping ourselves sane: A qualitative exploration of Black women's coping strategies for gendered racism. *Sex Roles, 82*, 512-524. https://doi.org/10.1007/s11199-019-01077-1

Stewart, E. A., Nicholson, W. K., Bradley, L., & Borah, B. J. (2013). The burden of uterine fibroids for African-American women: Results of a national survey. *Journal of Women's Health, 22*(10), 807-816. https://doi.org/10.1089/jwh.2013.4334

Watson, K. T., Roberts, N. M., & Saunders, M. R. (2012). Factors associated with anxiety and depression among African American and White women. *International Scholarly Research Notices, 2012*, Article 432321. https://doi.org/10.5402/2012/432321

West, L. M., Donovan, R. A., & Daniel, A. R. (2016). The price of strength: Black college women's perspectives on the strong Black woman stereotype. *Women & Therapy, 39*(3-4), 390-412. http://doi.org/10.1080/02703149.2016.1116871

ABOUT THE AUTHOR

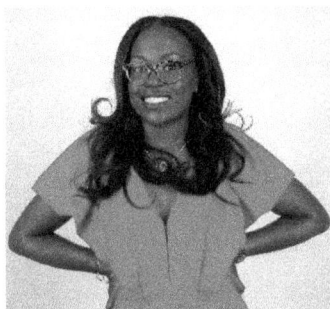

NA'TASHA EVANS, Ph.D.

**Educator | Research Scientist |
International Speaker | Author |
Philanthropist**

Dr. Na'Tasha Evans is a world-renowned educator, research scientist, international speaker, author, and philanthropist. She earned a Bachelor of Arts in Psychology, Bachelor of Science in Biology with a minor in Chemistry, and a Master of Education in Community Health from Cleveland State University. Further, she received a Doctorate in Health Education, with two graduate certificates in Patient Advocacy and Health Care Administration and Policy from the University of Toledo.

Dr. Evans is a Tenure-Track Assistant Professor of Health Education and Promotion in the School of Health Sciences for the College of Education, Health, and Human Services at Kent State University. Moreover, Dr. Evans is the Director of the Research and Education Collaborative for Health Disparities. Dr. Evans' research agenda focuses on examining health disparities and minority health, with an emphasis on examining maternal, child, and infant health; exploring patient-provider communication; and investigating women's health utilizing quantitative and qualitative methodological approaches. She has received national and international grants, worked with several community-based organizations, presented nationally and internationally, and published in peer-refereed journals. In addition to publishing in peer-refereed journals, Dr. Evans has authored several books, including *Inspire Me! Everything I Can Be from A to Z.*

Excited about educating and assisting others, Dr. Evans founded Inspired Minds Consulting Firm, LLC. The mission of Inspired Minds Consulting is to provide high-quality, comprehensive, and evidence-based research consulting; research training and professional development courses; thesis and dissertation coaching; and children's book coaching.

Always willing to give back, Dr. Evans has founded the Inspire Her Movement. The Inspire Her Movement provides hygiene kits to women and children in schools, group homes, shelters, and more.

www.ingramcontent.com/pod-product-compliance
Lightning Source LLC
Chambersburg PA
CBHW031447280326
41927CB00037B/389